Davina's
SMART CARBS

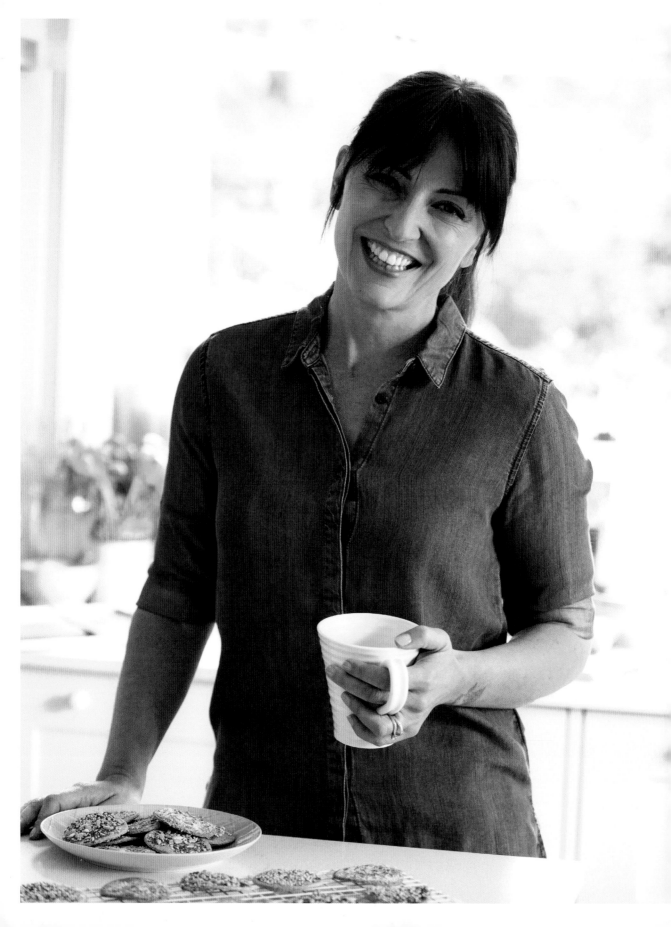

Davina's
SMART CARBS

Davina McCall

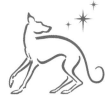

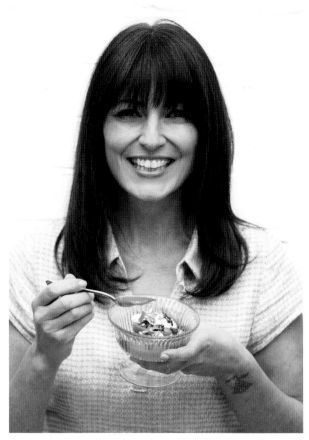

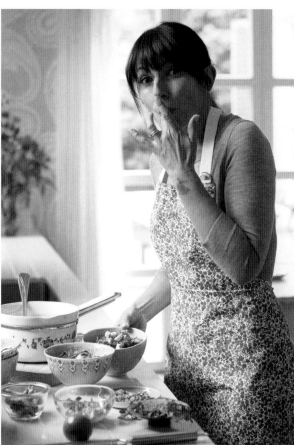

I would like to dedicate this book to my kids and ALL their friends. They inspire me to cook, to be healthy and they make me smile a lot! Also to Matthew for keeping me grounded . . . and running me baths in the evening. Lols . . . it's the little things (looking forward to growing old with you). Love you xxxxx

First published in Great Britain in 2015
by Orion Publishing Group Ltd
Carmelite House, 50 Victoria Embankment, London EC4Y 0DZ
An Hachette UK Company

10 9 8 7 6 5 4 3 2 1

Text © Davina McCall 2015
Design and layout © Orion 2015

A CIP catalogue record for this book is available from the British Library.

ISBN: 978 1 4091 5767 0

Designer: Paul Palmer-Edwards, Grade Design
Photographer: Andrew Hayes-Watkins
Art direction: Helen Ewing, Loulou Clark
Food director: Catherine Phipps
Food stylist: Anna Burges-Lumsden
Props stylist: Olivia Wardle
Project editor: Jinny Johnson
Proofreader: Elise See Tai
Indexer: Elizabeth Wiggans
Food stylist's assistants: Lou Kenny, Jane Brown

Nutritional advice and analysis: Fiona Hunter, Bsc (Hons) Nutrition, Dip Dietetics

Special thanks to Lakeland (www.lakeland.co.uk) for supplying cooking equipment for the photoshoots

Printed and bound in Germany

Note: While every effort has been made to ensure that the information in this book is correct, it should not be substituted for medical advice. The recipes in this book should be used in combination with a healthy lifestyle. If you are concerned about any aspect of your health, speak to your GP. People under medical supervision should not come off their medication without speaking to their health professional.

The Orion Publishing Group's policy is to use papers that are natural, renewable and recyclable products and made from wood grown in sustainable forests. The logging and manufacturing processes are expected to conform to the environmental regulations of the country of origin.

www.orionbooks.co.uk

For more delicious recipes, features, videos and exclusives from Orion's cookery writers, and to sign up for our 'Recipe of the Week' email visit **bybookorbycook.co.uk**

Contents

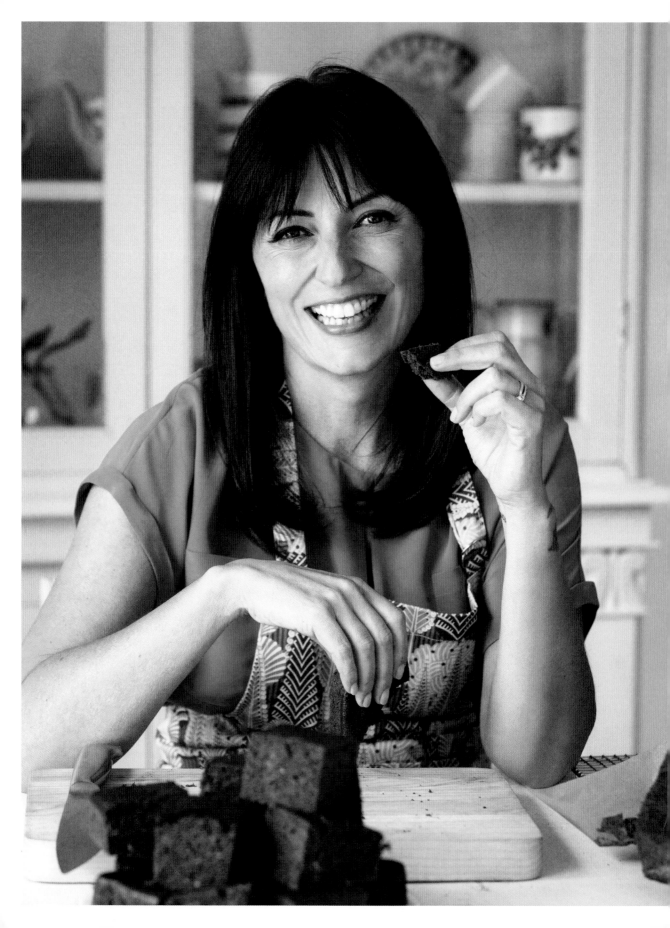

Loving the Smart Carbs

OMG, I am SO happy that you liked my *5 Weeks to Sugar-Free* cookbook. I love the fact that you all got the idea of sugar-free eating like I got it, and I ♡ hearing from you and seeing pics of the dishes you've made (they're looking good). And most important of all – people are realising that sugar-free doesn't mean pleasure-free. Keep it coming, gang.

While working on *Sugar-Free*, I realised there was a lot of confusion about carbohydrates. Mmmmm carbs... Lots of women were asking me about the benefits – or not – of carb-free diets, how to stop the carb cravings and ways to avoid those terrible carb slumps. They echoed my questions, so I set out to find the answers for us all.

Let's get one thing straight before we begin: I love carbs – crisps are my weakness – but I also know that the wrong ones do my body no good. And let's face it, we all work hard to stay in shape. So, is carb-free the answer? The experts say a resounding 'no'. Our bodies need carbs to work properly: we need them to look great, feel great, think straight and we need the fibre that carbs contain.

So how do we do it, how do we eat carbs and still look and feel fantastic? This book has the answer: smart carbs. I've worked with my amazing food team again to cut through the carb confusion and write recipes that work with real life, in real kitchens and for real appetites.

Smart carbs still have that great comfort-food feeling but they also provide us with loads of goodness and nutrients, as well as all-important fibre – and they're good for all the family. Going smart carb my way means eating lots of hearty soups and salads packed with veggies and pulses, snacking on home-made popcorn instead of crisps, enjoying yummy wholegrain bread instead of white sliced, and cooking up some sweet potato fries instead of chips. There's no added refined sugar and no junk in these recipes, and none of those dumb carbs that have loads of empty calories.

And along with your smart carbs, try my favourite protein-rich dishes, such as ricotta dumplings, Spanish chicken, slow-roast pork, seafood tagine, spinach and egg curry, or lamb and aubergine casserole. No deprivation here.

The aim of this book is to help you feed your body the good stuff and, if you follow my 5 week plan, you can achieve steady and healthy weight loss. You'll look and feel better, have more energy and avoid those mid-afternoon slumps. No way are you going to feel hungry. Smart carbs are the perfect fuel for your work-outs too.

I promise you – once you get into the smart carb habit you'll never want to stop.

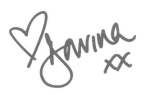

Carbs – the low-down

I admit it – I often crave carbs. I LOVE bread and couldn't bear to give it up so I've never liked the idea of a very low-carb diet. But when I started to think about the whole carb thing, I realised I needed to know more about carbs, why I long for them sometimes and how to tell the smart from the dumb.

To help me – and you – I fired lots of questions to my trusted nutrition expert to find out the truth about carbs. Are low-carb diets safe? Can I still eat bread? And why is it that sometimes I would swap everything I own for a doorstep slice of white toast with lashings of butter? Aargghhh! It's a minefield, but working out some great recipes to help us all choose the right kind of carbs – and lose weight – seemed just the right way to go. So here's the low-down.

Q: Some of my friends run screaming from carbs, but are they really that scary?

A: Not at all. Carbs are one of the three main food groups – the others are fat and protein – and they are important fuel for the body. Carbohydrates are contained in many types of food and our body uses them for energy – not only for the energy for running around and exercising but also the energy needed by our organs, including the brain, in order to work properly. Carbohydrates are broken down into simple sugar – glucose – which circulates in the bloodstream and is used by all the cells in the body.

Q: I guess that means it's not good to go too low-carb?

A: It's not. If you go too low you are depriving your body of important nutrients. It's never a good idea to cut out a whole food group. It's fine to cut down to a sensible level (see the 5 Week Plan on page 214) but instead of going low-carb, go SMART CARB!

Q: So some carbs are better for us than others?

A: Yes, there are different types of carbs: simple carbohydrates, such as table sugar, and complex carbohydrates, such as those found in grains, pulses and vegetables. Those are the ones to have.

Refined carbohydrates, such as white bread, white pasta and white rice, are digested quickly so they give us a rush of energy and a blood sugar spike. You're likely to get an equally speedy dip and you'll soon feel hungry again. Most of the good stuff, like dietary fibre, vitamins and minerals, has been stripped away from refined carbs, and sugar doesn't contain any nutrients at all.

What we need are complex carbs, as these are packaged with other nutrients. Complex carbs, such as unrefined wholegrains, pulses and vegetables, are digested more slowly, and so keep your blood sugar steady. And they contain plenty of vitamins and minerals.

Complex carbs contain fibre too, which makes you feel full for longer. When you are dieting you need to focus on foods like these that really pack a nutritional punch to help make sure you are getting all the vitamins and minerals you need. And it goes without saying that anything that helps you feel full and reduces the urge to snack has got to be a good thing.

Did you hear that people? Woop Woop!

BAD CARBS are refined and low in fibre. They are stripped of important vitamins and minerals and are bad news for blood sugar levels:

- White bread, pasta and rice
- Cakes and biscuits made with white flour and sugar
- Sweets
- Sweet fizzy drinks

GOOD CARBS contain fibre, vitamins and minerals and help keep blood sugar levels stable. They're the smart choice –they're SMART carbs:

- Root vegetables (except white potatoes)
- Pulses, such as beans, chickpeas and lentils
- Wholegrains, such as brown rice, oats, buckwheat, quinoa, rye, barley
- Whole fruit

SMART SWAPS

Crisps are my downfall. I can't resist them, but here's the good news – I love popcorn too and that is lower in carbohydrate and lower in calories. Don't go for the high-butter, high-sugar popcorn though. Make your own (see page 172 for my recipes). Here are some dumb/smart swap ideas:

DUMB CARB	SMART CARB
Cream cracker	Oatcake
Crisps	Popcorn
White potato	Sweet potato
Cornflakes	Porridge
Sweets/biscuits	Whole fruit
White rice	Brown rice
Couscous	Wholegrain couscous
White bread	Wholegrain/granary/rye bread

smart carbs ... totally delish AND filling!

Q: No reason why I can't enjoy the good carbs – smart carbs – then?

A: That's right. You don't want to cut out all carbs – you want to choose the right carbs, the carbs that contribute to a healthy, balanced diet and won't make you fat. Steer clear of dumb carbs – refined sugar, cakes, sweets, white bread and white pasta, sugary drinks – which are packed with calories but low in nutrition. Instead, go for vegetables, pulses and wholegrains.

Manufacturers add sugar and refined starch to processed foods and we really don't need those carbs. We need carbs that do something for us, that contain vitamins, minerals and fibre. These are 'smart carbs' and they are amazing.

Q: OK, this is all good, but why do I crave the bad carbs sometimes?

A: The thing about some carbs – the refined, white stuff – is that they are just so easy to eat. Think of that bread basket on the table in the restaurant, a packet of biscuits, a bag of crisps. When you're hungry they're all very tempting because they give you a quick lift. You can get through them in no time and before you know it, you've consumed loads of carbohydrate but done yourself no good at all. These carbs are quickly digested, giving you a surge of blood sugar, but all too soon you're hungry again. Then what do you want – more of those carbs! And that's what can make us fat.

Q: So are baguettes and chocolate bars out of my life for ever?

A: No, but make them something you treat yourself to very occasionally, and don't let them become a regular item on your menu. Make sure that most of what you eat contains smart carbs, packed with vitamins and minerals and fibre.

Q: Vitamins and minerals I know about, but remind me why we need fibre?

A: There's fibre in plant-based foods, such as veggies, wholegrains and fruit, and it's so important for our health. Not all fibre can be digested by the body. Some just passes through the system helping the bowels to work well – healthy poo, in other words. The other sort of fibre can be digested and is believed to help keep our cholesterol levels down. And because it is digested slowly it makes us feel full for longer and helps keep blood sugar levels steady – avoiding those energy dips and highs.

The latest report from an expert group known as Scientific Advisory Committee on Nutrition says that we all need to eat more fibre – the recommended amount for adults is 30g a day. Most of us manage less than half that. This new report also says that high-fibre diets are linked with a lower risk of stroke and heart disease, certain types of cancer and type 2 diabetes, the incidence of which has risen by 60 per cent in the last decade.

THESE ARE SOME HIGH-FIBRE FOODS:

- Lentils, beans and chickpeas
- Root veg, such as parsnips and carrots
- Green veg, such as broccoli and spinach
- Fruit, such as apples and pears
- Wholegrains, such as barley couscous and freekeh
- Quinoa
- Nuts and seeds

Q: And what can I have when I get that mid-afternoon energy slump?

A: That sluggish feeling in the afternoon is often a sign that the body is dehydrated. The first thing to do is to drink a large glass of water, then choose a healthy/smart carb snack like a handful of almonds, a piece of fruit or one of the snack recipes in this book. Some people do need to eat little and often. If you're one of them, you need to think ahead and make sure you've got smart snacks at hand so you don't get tempted by less healthy options.

Q: Will eating smart carbs help me lose weight?

A: When you're on a diet or watching your weight every calorie counts so you need to make sure your carbs work hard for you. In terms of health, food has to provide goodness – nutrients – so don't just focus on the calories. Good carbs take longer to digest but they keep you feeling fuller for longer because they contain fibre. They provide a steady supply of energy, not the spikes and falls you get with processed carbs.

Q: Can I eat any kind of veg?

A: Green vegetables such as broccoli, cabbage and so on are lowest in carbohydrates, but you can also eat starchy veg, such as sweet potatoes, carrots and squash, which contain lots of vitamins and minerals. The best idea is to have a good variety of seasonal veg, and then you get a great range of nutrients. Potatoes are not actually classified as a vegetable and although white potatoes do contain some vitamins and minerals and fibre, sweet potatoes are a smarter choice.

Q: And what about fruit?

A: Some people on very low-carb diets cut out all fruit, but that's not a good idea. Fruit contains loads of vitamins, minerals and other good stuff, such as phytochemicals, so it is really good for you. Best advice is to eat fruit in moderation – two or three portions a day. And eat a variety of fruit, not just one kind. It's true that berries, for example, are lower in calories, and have a lower GI, than tropical fruits such as mangos, but mangos are an excellent source of vitamins and of carotenes, both of which are important for health.

Always try to have the whole fruit, rather than just juice. Most of the fibre is removed from juice so it's quicker to digest – and much easier to have far too much of. You can easily gulp down the juice of six oranges, so taking in loads of sugar, but you're unlikely to eat six whole oranges all in one go.

Q: Do meat and fish contain carbs?

A: They don't. Red meat, poultry, fish and shellfish contain no carbohydrate and they are rich in protein, making them a good choice for anyone trying to lose weight. Watch out for processed meats, though, such as sausages and ham – most will contain some carb and/or sugar. Eggs and nuts are carb-free too.

Q: And dairy?

A: Milk, cheese and yoghurt all have some carbohydrate but they also contain fat, protein and lots of nutrients, like calcium which is really important for our bones. Avoid low-fat fruit or flavoured yoghurts, which have added sugar and can be surprisingly high in calories. Butter and oils do not contain carbs.

Q: Where do GI and GL come in? I've never quite managed to figure out what they're all about.

A: The glycaemic index, usually referred to as GI, measures the rate at which glucose from foods containing carbohydrates gets into the bloodstream. The faster the blood glucose level rises, the higher the GI of that food. In other words, foods with a high GI, like French bread, give you a quick glucose rush, but an equally quick slump. But certain things affect the GI of food, such as the cooking method and what the food is eaten with. So for example pasta, which is served al dente (still with a bit of bite to it) has a lower GI than pasta that is overcooked. A jacket potato, which by itself is high GI, is lower if served with baked beans.

Choose carbohydrates with a low to medium GI to keep your blood sugar levels stable. Some research also shows that low GI carbs help you feel full for longer so can help keep hunger pangs at bay. Examples of low GI foods include porridge oats, lentils and beans.

Then there is GL, or the glycaemic load, of a food. This is calculated by combining the GI and the amount of carbohydrate in a portion of food. Many nutritionists believe this is a more useful way of looking at the effect that carbs have on blood sugar. One of the things that it is important to understand is that size matters. Even when you are eating smart/low GI carbs you need to be mindful of the amount you are eating – particularly if you want to lose weight.

Q: What about my children? They need carbs don't they?

A: They do, but like the rest of us they're better off with smart carbs. Get your children off to a healthy start by encouraging them to eat unprocessed, nutritional food, with plenty of fibre. When they're growing fast they might need extra calories, so offer extra veg, wholegrain bread with their meals and snacks such as peanut butter on oatcakes. Help them make good food choices right from the start.

Q: And what about when I'm working out? I need carbs – will I have enough while I'm on the 5 week plan?

The recipes in this book contain enough smart carbs to fuel your workouts. Have a look at the meal planner at the back to help you choose your meals and healthy snacks. Before a workout you need something light and easy to digest, such as yoghurt with a couple of spoonfuls of muesli, or a couple of oatcakes with red pepper dip (see page 155) or some roasted chickpeas (see page 173). After a workout you need a combination of slow- and quick-release carbs – a banana and glass of milk is ideal. A glass of milk is better than many sports drinks because it not only helps to rehydrate the body but also provides protein to repair muscle and electrolytes, which are lost when you exercise.

Healthy plate

This is roughly how the contents of your plate should look for most meals:

50 per cent salad or vegetables

25 per cent lean protein
(such as lean meat, poultry or fish)

25 per cent smart carbs

How many cals?

Carbs, fat and protein all give us energy but in different amounts:

- Carbs: about 4 kcal per gram
- Protein: about 4 kcal per gram
- Fat: about 9 kcal per gram

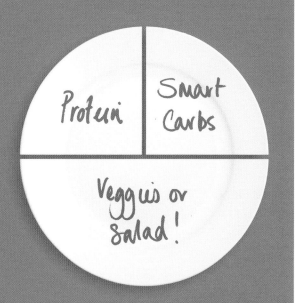

A FEW COOKING NOTES

(F) Lots of the recipes can be frozen so look out for the freezer symbol.

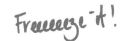

Garlic, onions and other veg are to be peeled unless otherwise specified. The weights given in the ingredient lists are the peeled weight.

Stock isn't hard to make and we had a recipe for chicken stock in *5 Weeks to Sugar-Free*, but there are plenty of good ready-made fresh stocks available in supermarkets now.

I like to use free-range chicken and eggs whenever I can but that's up to you.

My eating plan – eat smart and lose weight

I'm loving smart carbs and I'm so excited about the recipes in this book. As well as fab main dishes like chicken curry, tuna pasta and beef casserole, I've included loads of wonderful soups and salads and healthy snacks, such as roasted chickpeas, oatcakes, smoky almonds and lots of kinds of popcorn. I could never give up bread and I have a recipe for a fabulous walnut and rye loaf – made with wholegrains. It is sooooo good. And you have to try my amazing lasagne made with tortilla wraps instead of pasta. You won't believe how light and dreamy it is. There are even some puds and bakes. Like the sound of chocolate panna cotta? Sticky toffee pudding? Hobby nobby biscuits?

The aim of this book is not to banish carbs but to reduce your carb intake to a sensible level – and make sure all those carbs are smart carbs. These are not crazy unrealistic recipes that demand all sorts of weird things and that the rest of your family might not enjoy. It's all normal family-friendly food, but containing smart carbs and lots of fibre. If you follow my 5 week plan at the back of the book you will gradually reduce your carb intake while still eating enough to keep your body running well. And the family will be happy too.

All the recipes in this book contain only smart carbs – apart from a little honey and maple syrup in the puds – so you don't need to worry. We've made the decisions for you.

Calories – to count or not to count?

Lots of you have told me that you like calorie-counted diets and you want more calorie info so that's what we're doing in this book. There are calorie counts on each page – and there's full nutritional info for each recipe in the back, telling you how much carb, fat, protein and sugar there is in each recipe.

Everyone says that very strict calorie-counted diets are not a good idea. They're hard to stick to, you feel deprived and the minute you fall off the wagon you tend to eat more than usual and put on the weight you lost and then some.

But to lose weight you do need to spend more energy than you take in. If you follow my 5 week plan you'll drop from 1,400 to 1,200 calories a day. That's easy to do, you won't feel hungry and you'll have enough energy to exercise.

What's in my book

- Easy recipes for family meals packed with smart carbs and goodness.
- Nothing too complicated and all the ingredients are available in supermarkets.
- No refined white carbs or refined sugar in anything, but there are a few puds and cakes made with maple syrup or honey for that occasional treat.
- A 5 week eating plan to help you gradually reduce calories to a level for steady weight loss.

I'm loving all these recipes so hope you do too.
Good luck and lots of love

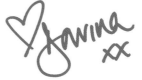

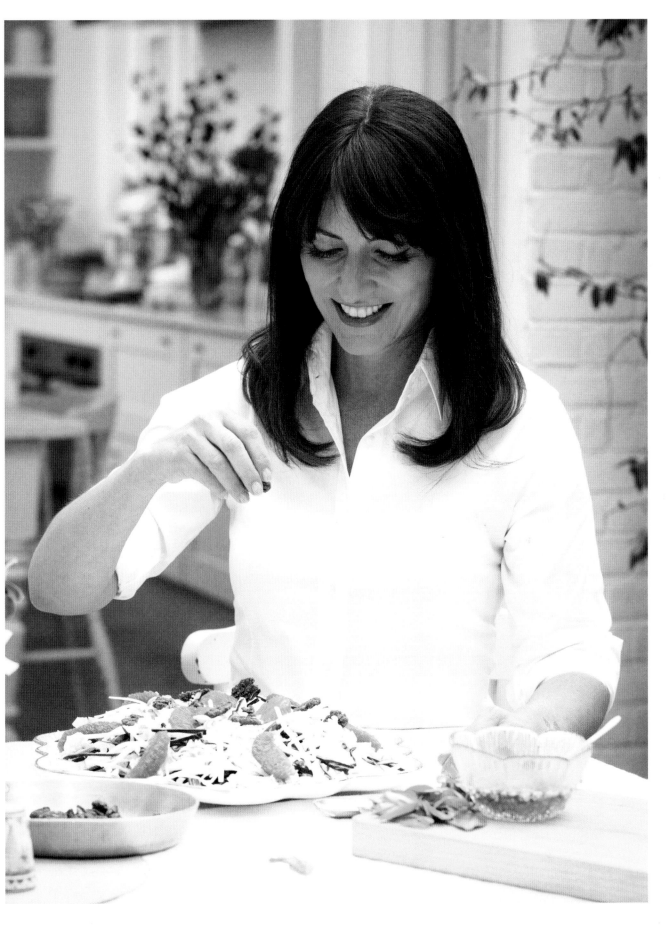

My Faves

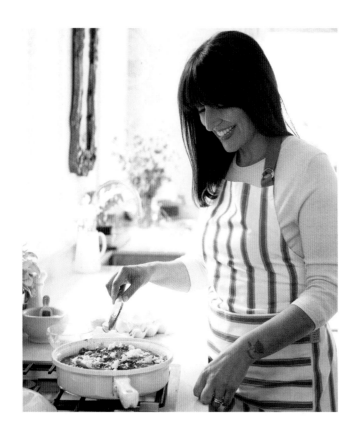

Chapter 1

Brunch + Light Bites

"Great smart carbs start to the day
– or at any time."

Buckwheat blinis

Blinis are easy to make, but you do need to think ahead and allow time for the batter to rest. For a really special brunch, serve the blinis with lots of smoked salmon and some crème fraiche – SO good.

1 Put the flours, yeast and salt in a large bowl and mix them together thoroughly. Warm the milk very gently in a saucepan, just to take the chill off it, then pour it into a bowl and whisk in the yoghurt and egg yolks. Add the milk mixture to the dry ingredients and stir thoroughly to combine. Cover the bowl with cling film or a damp cloth and leave the batter to stand for an hour and a half. It will stay quite liquid, but lots of little air bubbles will appear.

2 Whisk the egg whites in a bowl until they form stiff peaks. Fold a large tablespoon of the egg whites into the batter to loosen it a little, then add the rest. Leave the batter to rest for another hour.

3 When you're ready to cook the blinis, heat a big frying pan and spray it with oil. Drop spoonfuls of the batter into the frying pan and flatten them slightly. As soon as bubbles appear on top of the blinis and the undersides are cooked, flip them over and cook on the other side. They'll need about a minute on each side.

4 Serve the blinis while they're still slightly warm, topped with crème fraiche, smoked salmon and a sprinkling of chopped chives. A squeeze of lemon juice is essential too.

5 The blinis will keep for a few days. To refresh them, wrap them in foil and warm them through in a moderate oven. They also freeze well.

Makes about 16

100g buckwheat flour
50g wholemeal or wholemeal
 spelt flour
½ tsp instant dried yeast
½ tsp salt
150ml whole milk
100ml plain yoghurt
2 eggs, separated
olive oil spray

To serve
crème fraiche
smoked salmon
finely chopped chives
squeeze of lemon juice

60 calories per blini

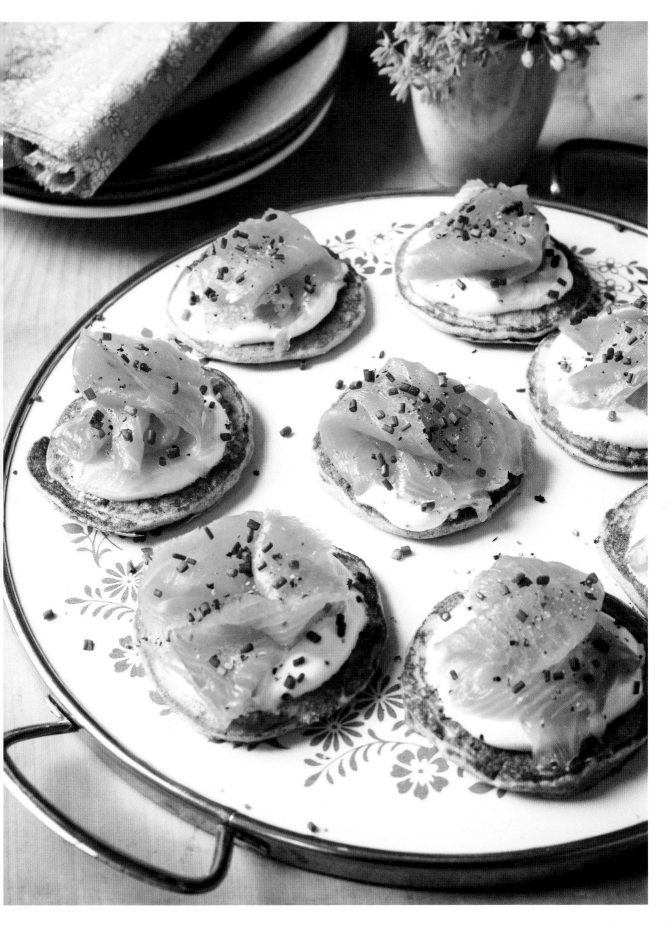

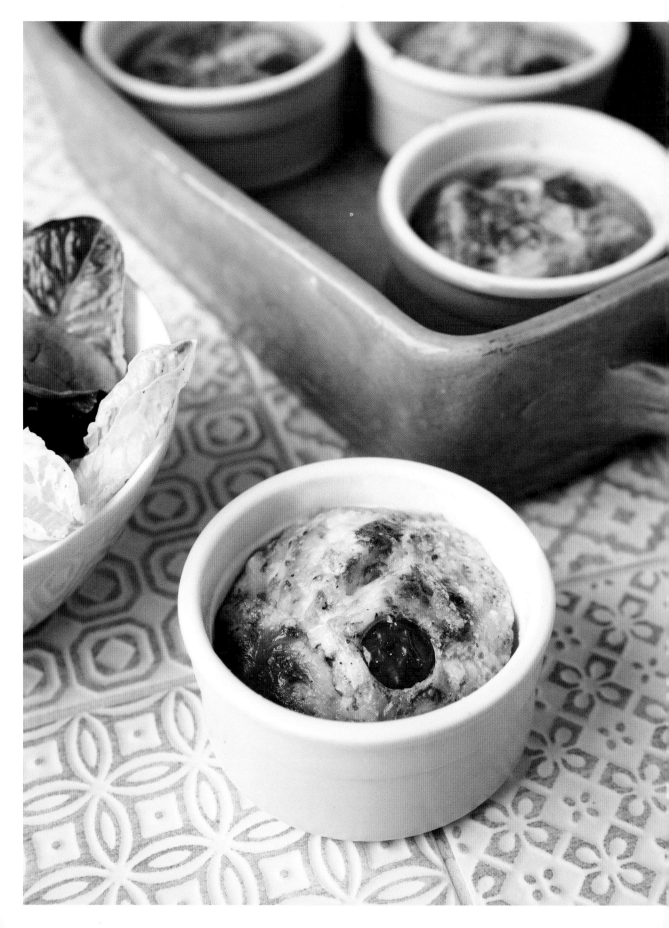

Pastryless quiches

I love all things eggy and quiches are a big fave, but I don't like eating lots of carb-heavy pastry. We came up with this brilliant solution – a quiche-type filling baked in little ramekins so no need for pastry. Lovely with a green salad on the side. If you include the cheese it adds another 25 calories per quiche. P.S. Have I mentioned that I like eggs?

1 Preheat the oven to 180°C/160°C Fan/Gas 4. Spray the insides of the ramekins with oil or grease them with a little butter.

2 Crack the eggs into a large bowl and beat them to combine. Whisk the milk and crème fraiche together in a separate bowl, then add them to the eggs. Whisk the mixture until it's smooth, but don't let it get too frothy. Season with salt and pepper, then add the herbs and the grated cheese, if using.

3 Put a cherry tomato in the centre of each ramekin and pour in the egg mixture, dividing it evenly between the dishes. Place the ramekins in a roasting dish or tin and pour in enough just-boiled water to come two-thirds of the way up the sides. Bake the quiches in the oven for 20–25 minutes. There should still be a slight wobble in the centre of each one.

4 If you are planning to turn the quiches out on to plates, leave them to stand for a few minutes so they will pop out easily. Otherwise, serve them immediately in the ramekins.

Serves 4

olive oil spray or butter
4 eggs
1 tbsp milk
50ml crème fraiche
1 tbsp finely chopped parsley
1 tbsp finely chopped chervil
1 tbsp finely chopped tarragon
25g hard cheese, such as Manchego, Gruyère or mature Cheddar, grated (optional)
4 cherry tomatoes
salt and black pepper

170 calories per serving; 195 with cheese

Bubble and squeak

Everyone loves this dish (especially Matthew) and it makes a brill brunch with some eggs. You can, of course, make it with any leftovers, but otherwise cook the vegetables in advance and let them cool thoroughly before making your bubble.

1 Bring a saucepan of water to the boil. Add the carrots and swede and cook them for about 10 minutes or until tender. Drain them thoroughly, then tip them back into the saucepan and leave them over a low heat for a few minutes, just to help steam off any excess liquid. Swede in particular can get quite waterlogged, so this is important.

2 Mash the carrots and swede with the butter until fairly smooth. Tip the mash into a bowl and leave it to cool, then chill it in the fridge for a while to firm it up.

3 Wash the greens thoroughly, put them in a saucepan with a little water and cover the pan. Place the pan over the heat and cook for a few minutes until the greens have wilted down, then drain them thoroughly and leave them to cool.

4 When you're ready to cook the bubble and squeak, mix the root veg mash and the greens together and season them with salt and pepper.

5 Heat the oil in a large non-stick frying pan and gently fry the chopped onion over a medium heat until it's softened and caramelising around the edges. Add this to the vegetables, then tip everything back into the frying pan and spread the mixture out into a large round. Cook the bubble and squeak over a medium heat for several minutes until it's nice and brown underneath and cooked through.

6 Meanwhile, preheat your grill to its highest setting. Spritz the top of the bubble and squeak with olive oil spray, then pop it under the grill for 3–4 minutes until it's browning around the edges and in patches on top. Cut it into wedges and serve as part of a brunch with poached or fried eggs if you like.

Serves 4

300g carrots, cut into chunks
300g swede, cut into chunks
10g butter
150g spring greens, cabbage or
    Brussels sprouts, shredded
1 tbsp olive oil
1 small onion, finely chopped
olive oil spray
poached or fried eggs (optional)
salt and black pepper

119 calories per serving; 193 with poached egg; 211 with fried egg

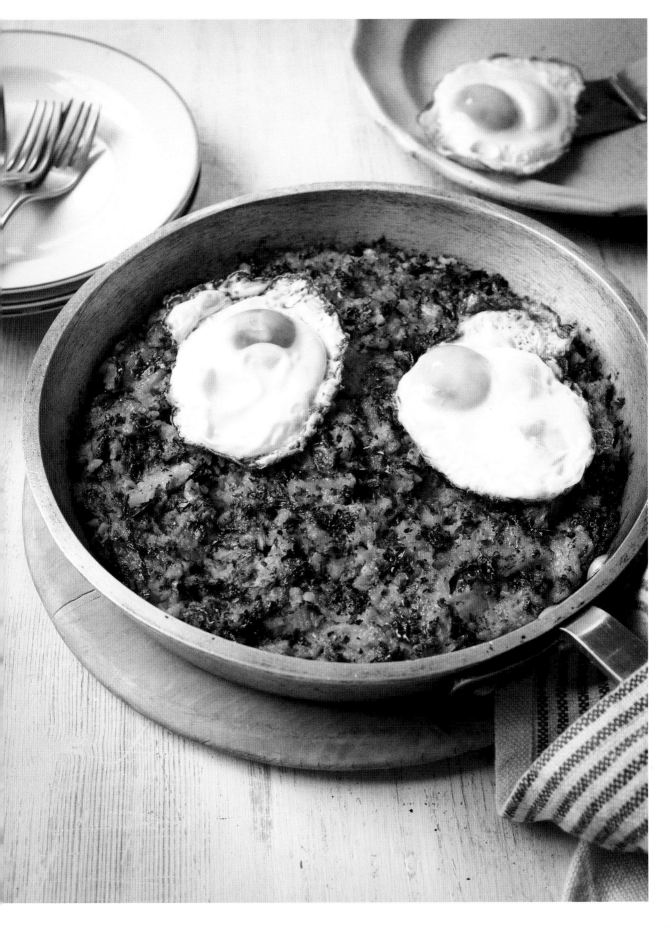

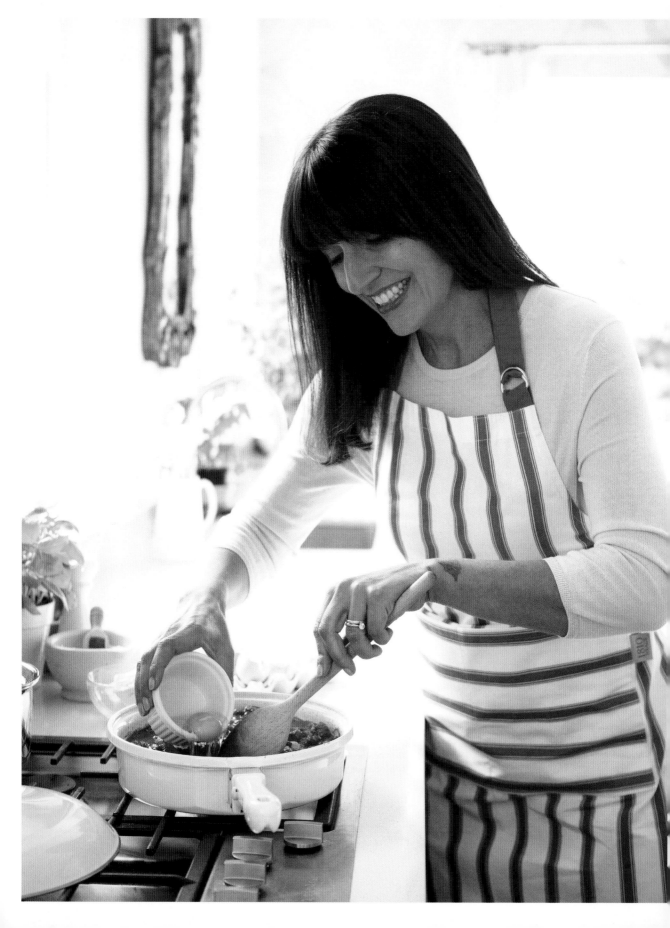

Veggie shakshuka (a sort of ratatouille with eggs)

The name of this scared me off at first, but it's really just lovely veg with eggs – easy peasy. I'm happy to eat this at any time of day but it makes a brilliant brunch. And if you're really organised you could make the pepper and tomato mixture the night before so getting the dish on the table is a doddle. Good served with the chickpea flatbreads on page 156.

1 Heat the olive oil in a large, straight-sided frying pan (you need one with a lid), then add the red onion, peppers and celery. Stir them for a minute or so, then turn down the heat, cover the pan and leave the veggies to cook for about 5 minutes. Add the garlic, cumin and cinnamon, stir for another minute or so, then add the tomatoes. Season with salt and pepper, taste and add the honey if the tomatoes are particularly sharp.

2 Cover the pan again and simmer for another 10 minutes until the vegetables have softened but still keep their shape – at this stage you can set the pan aside for a while if you're preparing things in advance. Otherwise, take the lid off the pan and simmer the veg for another 5 minutes, then stir in the herbs.

3 Make 4 little dips in the sauce and drop an egg into each one. Sprinkle some crumbled feta over each egg, then cover the pan. Cook over a very low heat for a few more minutes until the egg whites have just set and the yolks are still runny. The feta should protect the yolks from getting overcooked. Serve immediately.

Serves 4

1 tbsp olive oil
1 red onion, thinly sliced
2 red peppers, thinly sliced
2 celery sticks, sliced
1 garlic clove, finely chopped
1 tsp cumin seeds
pinch of cinnamon
2 x 400g cans of chopped
    tomatoes
1 tsp honey (optional)
small bunch of coriander
    or parsley, finely chopped
4 eggs
50g feta cheese, crumbled
salt and black pepper

215 calories per serving

Beans and eggs

A nice brunch or lunch dish. This has a lovely smoky mellow flavour, but if you want to spice things up, add some chilli or put a bottle of hot sauce on the table so everyone can help themselves. You can top it with fried eggs instead of poached if you like, but that will add a few extra calories.

1 Heat the olive oil in a large shallow frying pan that has a lid. Add the smoked bacon and cook for several minutes until it's all well browned, stirring regularly. Add the onions and red pepper, then cook for another 5 minutes over a medium heat until the vegetables are starting to brown slightly round the edges.

2 Add the garlic, oregano, beans, coconut milk and lime zest, then season with salt and pepper. Cook for 5 minutes over a medium heat, uncovered, to allow the sauce to reduce a little, then add the broccoli. Cover the pan and cook for another 6–7 minutes over a low heat until the broccoli is tender. Add half the lime juice and taste, then add more if you think it is necessary.

3 Serve the beans sprinkled with coriander leaves and topped with poached eggs.

P.S. The coconut milk makes this taste crazy amazing.

Serves 4 beans only

1 tbsp olive oil
100g smoked bacon, chopped
2 medium red onions, diced
1 red pepper, diced
2 garlic cloves, finely chopped
½ tsp dried oregano
2 x 400g cans of black-eyed beans, drained and rinsed (about 500g drained weight)
400ml can of coconut milk
zest and juice of 1 lime
200g tenderstem or sprouting broccoli, cut into 3cm lengths
salt and black pepper

To serve
fresh coriander leaves
4 poached eggs

522 calories per serving

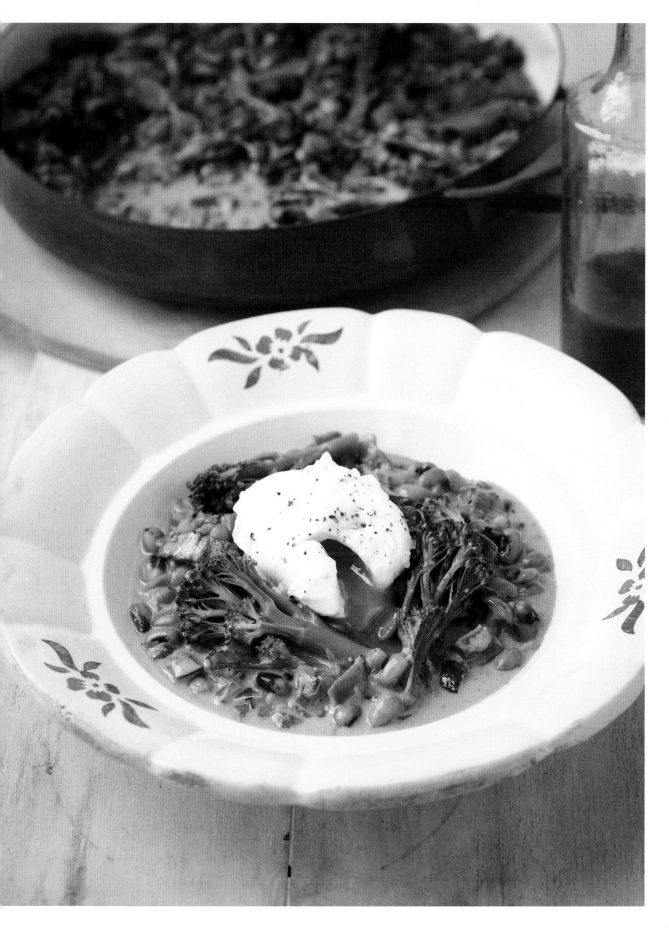

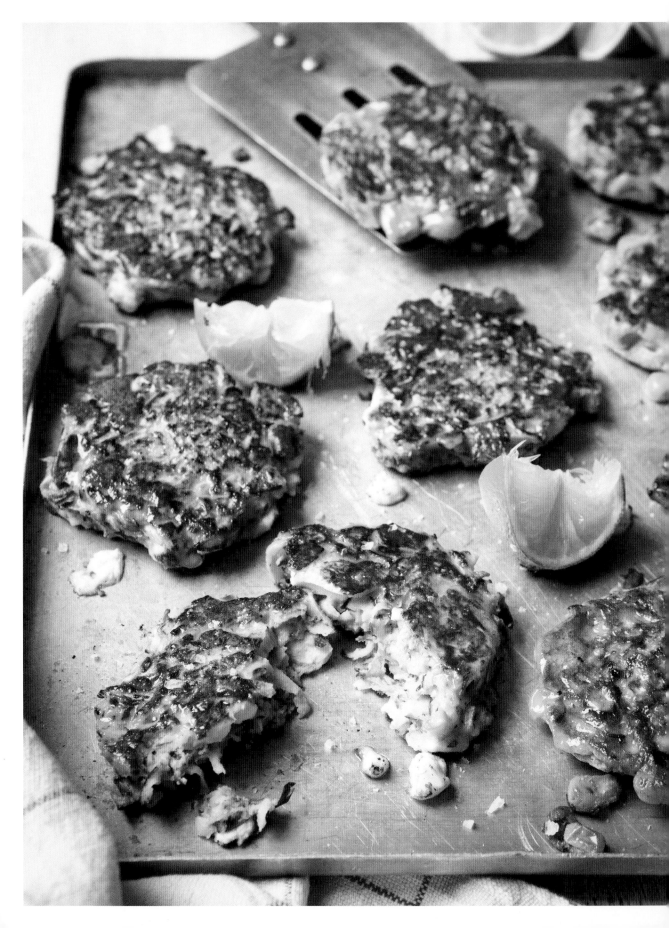

Fritters

I love a fritter and these are fab at any time of day. I like to make both kinds and let everyone help themselves to their favourites. I find that frozen corn works best – the kernels seem bigger and juicier – so I always keep a bagful in the freezer. Chickpea flour works well for these and you can buy it in supermarkets.

Sweetcorn fritters

1 Put the flour in a large bowl and make a well in the middle. Mix together the egg yolk and soy sauce, pour this mixture into the well, then gradually whisk it into the flour until you have a fairly firm batter.

2 Fold the sweetcorn kernels, spring onions and chopped coriander into the batter and mix thoroughly. Whisk the egg white in a bowl until it forms soft peaks. Add a tablespoon of this to the sweetcorn mixture to loosen it slightly, then as gently as possible, fold the rest of the egg white into the batter with a metal spoon.

3 Heat a teaspoon of oil in a large frying pan and keep it over a medium to high heat. Drop dessertspoonfuls of the batter into the frying pan and flatten them with the back of the spoon. You should be able to cook about 5–6 fritters at a time. Cook the fritters for a minute or so on each side until golden brown. Keep the first batch warm in a low oven while you cook the rest, then serve immediately.

Makes about 16

50g chickpea (gram) flour
    or wholemeal flour
1 egg, separated
2 tbsp light soy sauce
300g sweetcorn kernels,
    defrosted
2 spring onions, finely chopped
2 tbsp finely chopped coriander
    leaves (optional)
1–2 tbsp olive oil

37 calories per fritter

Courgette and feta fritters

1 Put the grated courgette in a colander lined with kitchen paper and leave it to drain. Take handfuls of courgette and squeeze out as much water from it as you can.

2 Put the flour in a large bowl and season it with salt and pepper. Make a well in the middle and add the eggs, then whisk them into the flour until you have a smooth batter. Add the courgettes, feta, herbs, lime zest and paprika, if using, to the batter and stir thoroughly to make a fairly wet mixture.

3 Heat a teaspoon of oil in a big frying pan. Add large tablespoons of the batter and flatten them with the back of the spoon. You should be able to cook 4 at a time. Cook the fritters on one side for 1–2 minutes until the batter has set and is a deep golden brown. Flip and cook the other side, then keep them warm in a low oven while you cook the next batch. Serve with wedges of lime and some crème fraiche if you like.

Makes about 20

500g courgettes, grated
85g chickpea (gram) flour
2 eggs, beaten
150g feta cheese, crumbled
1 tsp dried mint
2 tbsp finely chopped basil
    leaves
zest of 1 lime
½ tsp smoked paprika (optional)
1–2 tbsp olive oil
salt and black pepper

53 calories per fritter

Ricotta dumplings

I'd never heard of these until quite recently, but I'm so glad I have now. The proper Italian name for them is gnudi, and they're like little ricotta dumplings and are incredibly delish. I know 'dumpling' sounds heavy, but trust me – these are beautifully light and fluffy. Serve them with a fresh tomato sauce or a more traditional butter and sage sauce. The gnudi do need to chill for eight hours before cooking so it's best to prepare them the day before. They make a lovely starter or little lunch.

1 Strain the ricotta into a bowl, discarding any liquid, then add the Parmesan and a light grating of nutmeg. Season with salt and pepper, then mix thoroughly until smooth.

2 Cover a tray or a large plate with semolina. Wet your hands, then dip them into the semolina and take a heaped teaspoon of the ricotta mixture. Shape it into a ball or a flatter round patty, as you like, then drop it into the semolina. You could also use a couple of spoons to make oval shapes if you like. You should be able to make about 20 little dumplings with this mixture.

3 When you've shaped all your gnudi, sprinkle over more semolina so they are completely covered. Put them into the fridge to chill for at least 8 hours, or overnight.

4 When you are ready to cook, gently remove each dumpling from the semolina, patting off any excess, then put them on a plate. Bring a large saucepan of salted water to the boil. Turn the heat down to a simmer, then drop in all the gnudi and leave them to cook.

5 The gnudi are ready when they float to the top – this should take 3–4 minutes. Serve them in warm bowls with your chosen sauce.

Fresh tomato sauce

Heat the olive oil in a frying pan and add the garlic. Cook for a few moments, then add the tomatoes. Immediately remove the pan from the heat, add the sage leaves and lemon zest, then season the tomatoes with salt and pepper. Leave to stand while you cook the gnudi.

Butter sauce

Heat the butter in a frying pan and allow it to brown very lightly. Add the shredded sage and lemon zest and season with salt and pepper. Swirl round a few times, then pour the sauce over the gnudi.

Serves 4

300g ricotta cheese, drained
30g Parmesan cheese, finely grated
grating of fresh nutmeg
250g semolina, for sprinkling
salt and black pepper

Fresh tomato sauce
2 tbsp olive oil
1 garlic clove, finely chopped
500g very ripe fresh tomatoes, chopped
fresh sage leaves
zest of 1 lemon

Butter sauce
25g butter
several sage leaves, finely shredded
zest of 1 lemon

436 calories per serving with fresh tomato sauce; 412 with butter sauce

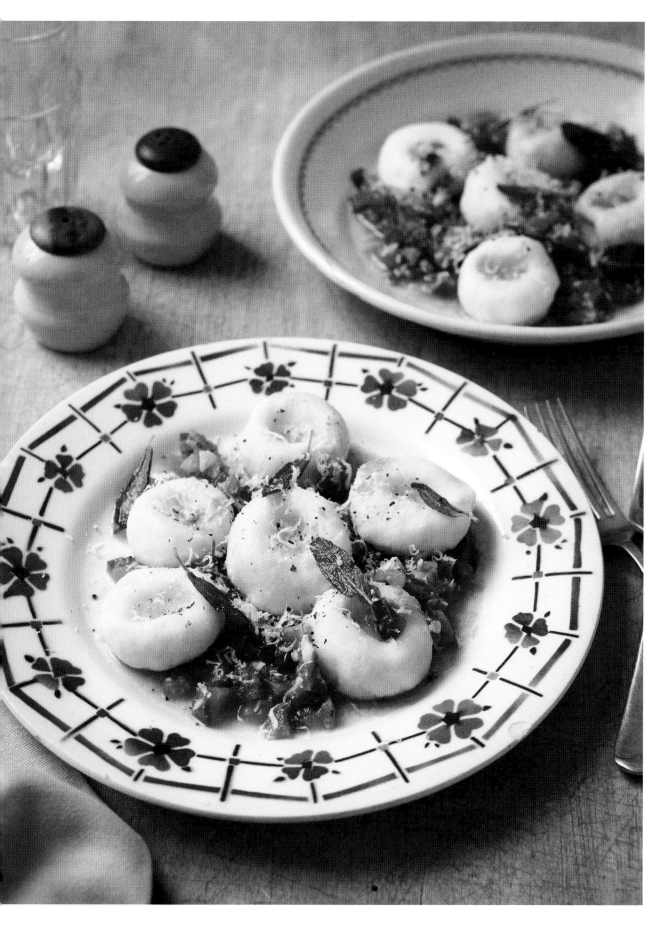

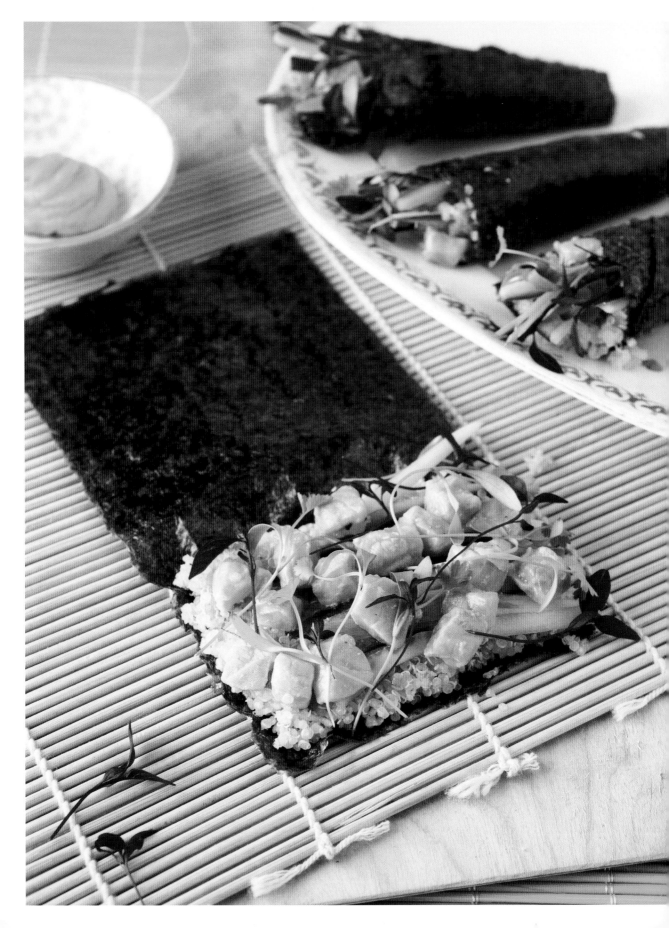

Salmon hand rolls

Amazing! Sushi made with quinoa is such a brilliant idea. I'd never made any sushi-type things at home before, but these are so easy. Best to make them just before you want to eat though, as they can go a bit soggy if you leave them for too long. You can add avocado too if you like and you don't mind the extra calories. BTW, nori is a kind of seaweed and you can buy it in supermarkets now. Great show-off meal for mates.

1 Dice the salmon into ½cm cubes and season them with salt and pepper. Mix the lime juice and soy sauce together and pour it over the salmon. Turn the salmon gently until all the cubes are lightly coated with lime and soy, then set them aside for a few moments.

2 Put the quinoa in a bowl, season it with salt and pepper and stir in the orange juice.

3 Cut each square of nori in half, following the straight lines. Place a half sheet in your hand, with a short side running along the wrist end of your palm. Put a heaped tablespoon of quinoa over the third of the nori sheet closest to you and spread evenly. Sprinkle over the cucumber, spring onions and cress or herbs, placing them high enough so that they will poke out a little once rolled. Finally, add a quarter of the salmon fillet.

4 To roll, take the corner closest to you and fold it up to the top corner where the filling ends. Then simply wrap the rest of the nori sheet round until you have an ice cream cone shape. Serve with pickled ginger, wasabi or chilli sauce, if you like. Eat immediately.

Serves 4

100g skinned salmon fillet, well chilled
juice of ½ lime
1 tsp light soy sauce
120g cooked quinoa (see p.204), cooled (or use ready-cooked)
2 tbsp freshly squeezed orange juice
2 pieces of sushi nori
6cm chunk of cucumber, cut into thin strips, lengthways
2 spring onions, finely sliced into long strips
cress, chives or other herbs
salt and black pepper

To serve
sushi pickled ginger
wasabi paste
chilli sauce such as sriracha (optional)

124 calories per serving

Citrus chilli fish

This is a version of the Latin American dish ceviche, which I've seen on loads of menus but never made myself. Would you believe it is so easy? It's really just fish 'cooked' in a marinade and served with a little salad. You could add diced avocado to the salad if you're a fan like me. Yaaay!

1 First make the marinade. Combine all the ingredients in a bowl and leave them to stand for 10 minutes. Strain and reserve the liquid.

2 Soak the slices of onion in cold water for 5 minutes – this makes their flavour milder. Peel the oranges and divide them into segments.

3 Using a sharp knife and cutting on the diagonal, slice the fish into thin strips of about 3 x 1cm – this is much easier to do if the fish is well chilled. Put the strips of fish in a shallow dish, sprinkle them with salt and leave them for 2 minutes, then pour over the marinade. Stir gently to combine, then set the fish aside for 2 minutes – no longer.

4 Dry the onions thoroughly. Arrange them on 4 plates, with the orange segments, then strain the fish from the marinade and divide the strips between the plates. Drizzle over a little of the marinade and serve sprinkled with coriander leaves and chilli.

Serves 4

600g sea bass, or other firm white
   fish, filleted, skinned and chilled
salt

Marinade
juice of 4 limes
10g piece of fresh root ginger, finely
   chopped
2 garlic cloves, finely chopped
1 red chilli, finely chopped
pinch of salt

To serve
½ red onion, finely sliced
2 oranges
sprigs of fresh coriander
1 red chilli, deseeded and finely
   chopped

282 calories per serving

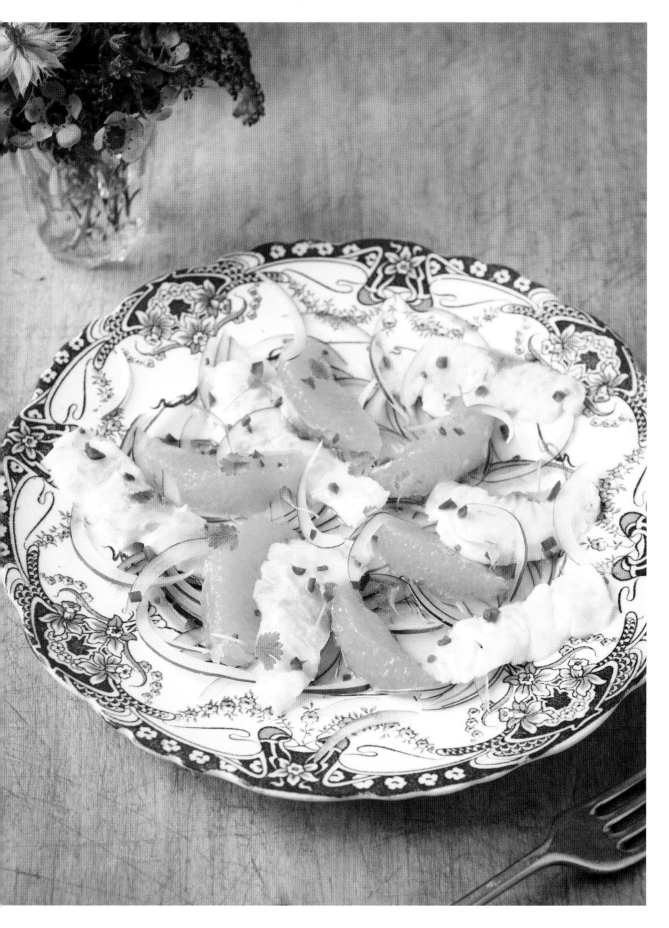

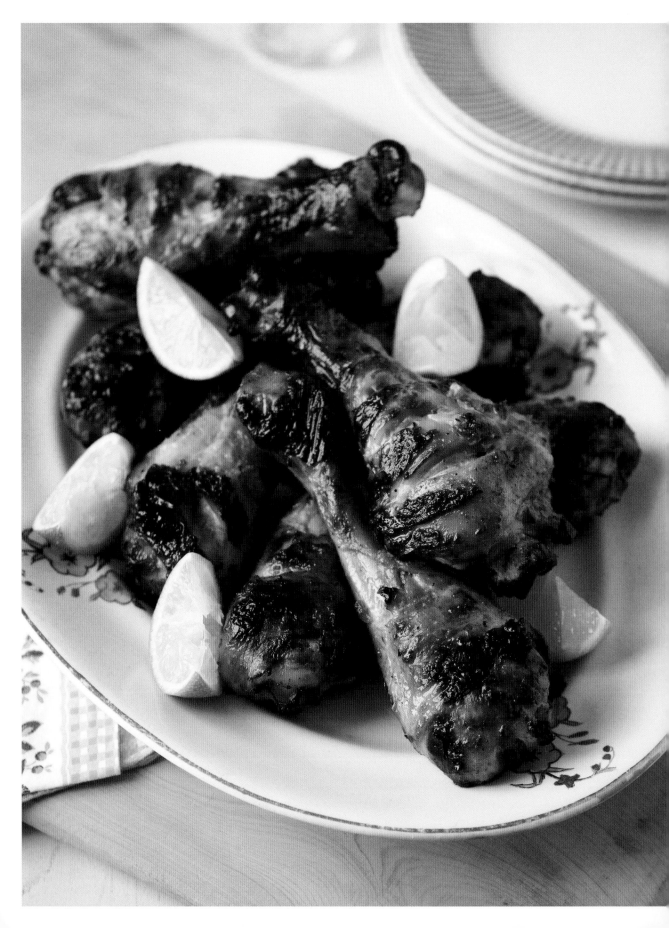

Buttermilk chicken

I think drumsticks are perfect for this as they are cheap to buy and my kids love them, but you can use any chicken pieces you like. The chicken is uncoated – no flour or breadcrumbs – to keep the carbs down, but still yummy and really easy to prepare. Just remember to allow time for the marinating. I promise there is nothing difficult about buttermilk and you can buy it in most supermarkets.

1 Slash the skin of the drumsticks a few times to allow the marinade to penetrate. Mix the buttermilk with the paprika, garlic and lime zest and season it with the salt and freshly ground pepper. Pour the buttermilk mixture over the chicken and massage it in. Leave the chicken to marinate in the fridge for at least 3 hours, but preferably overnight.

2 Remove the chicken from the fridge a good half an hour before you want to cook it so it can come to room temperature. Preheat the oven to 220°C/200°C Fan/Gas 7.

3 Line a baking tray with foil. Scrape any excess marinade off the pieces of chicken and arrange them evenly on the tray. Roast the chicken drumsticks in the oven for about 30 minutes, until they are all well browned and preferably slightly blackened in places. Serve with wedges of lime to squeeze over them.

Serves 4

8 chicken drumsticks, skin on
284ml carton of buttermilk
1 tsp sweet smoked paprika
2 garlic cloves, crushed
zest of 1 lime
1 tsp salt
1 tsp freshly ground black pepper
lime wedges, to serve

262 calories per serving

Pork sliders and quick apple coleslaw

A really yummy, lower-calorie version of a burger. Win win! You can bake or griddle these little sliders – whatever you find easiest. I like to serve them on lettuce leaves, but kids and non-dieters might prefer buns and you can add slices of tomato, onion rings and so on as you like. The smoky flavours of the pork are perfect with the apple coleslaw.

1 If you're going to bake the sliders, preheat the oven to 220°C/200°C Fan/Gas 7. Put the pork mince in a bowl with the oregano, garlic, mustard powder, fennel seeds, breadcrumbs or quinoa, egg and milk. Season with salt and pepper, then mix thoroughly – it's easiest to do this with your hands.

2 Divide the mixture into 8 patties and flatten them very slightly. Place the sliders on a baking tray and bake them in the oven for about 15 minutes. Alternatively, spray a large frying pan or griddle with oil and fry or grill the sliders for 4–5 minutes on each side until they're charred and cooked through.

3 Leave the sliders to rest for a few minutes. Place each one on a lettuce leaf, add a spoonful of coleslaw and top with another lettuce leaf. Add slices of tomato and/or red onion if you like.

Quick apple coleslaw

To make the apple coleslaw, mix the grated apple with the spring onions and cabbage and season with salt. Whisk the cider vinegar with the crème fraiche or yoghurt, and the mustard, if using, then stir this mixture into the apple and cabbage. If necessary, drain the coleslaw slightly before serving with the sliders.

Serves 4   sliders only (F)

500g pork mince
1 tsp dried oregano
1 garlic clove, crushed
½ tsp mustard powder
½ tsp fennel seeds, lightly crushed
100g wholemeal breadcrumbs or cooked quinoa (see p.204)
1 egg
25ml whole milk
olive oil spray (optional)
lettuce leaves
slices of tomato and onion (optional)
salt and black pepper

Quick apple coleslaw
1 green apple, peeled and grated
4 spring onions, finely chopped
¼ small green or white cabbage, finely shredded
1 tsp cider vinegar
1 tbsp crème fraiche or yoghurt
½ tsp Dijon or American mustard (optional)

337 calories per serving

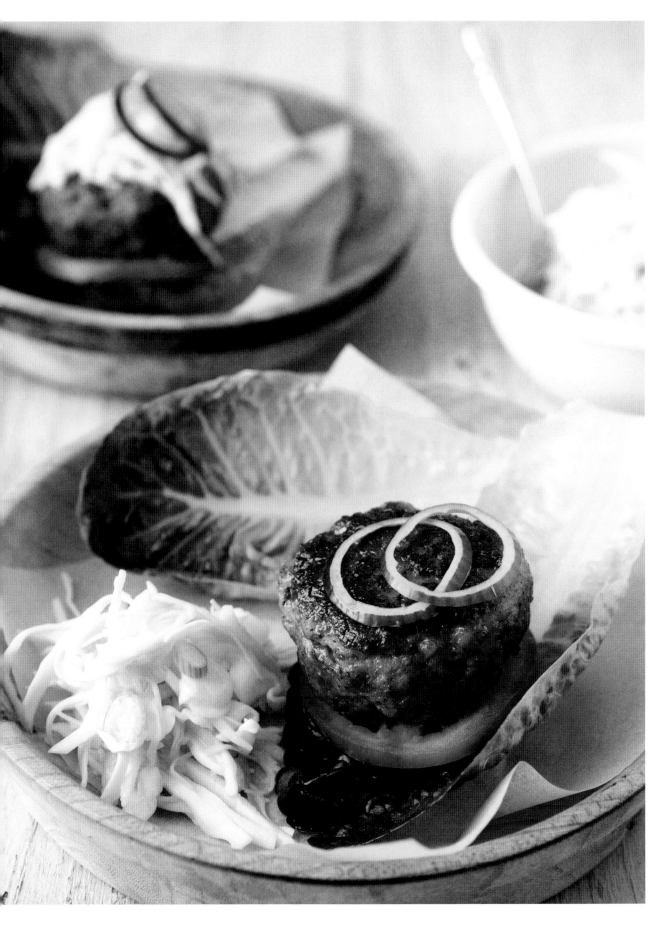

My Faves

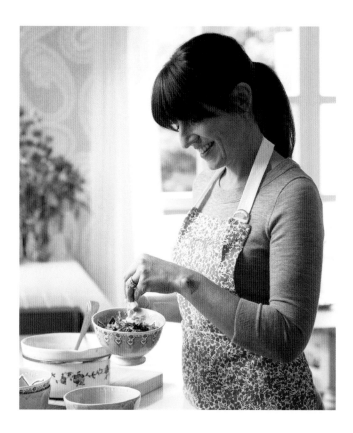

Chapter 2

Soups

"Nothing like a good soup:
filling and warming, nourishing
and comforting."

Carrot, celeriac and coriander soup

A bit of butter really does boost the flavour of this soup but if you prefer, you can use a tablespoon of olive oil instead of the butter and oil combo. A mild stock is best, so you don't overpower the veg, or you can use just water. I like the feta garnish – but then I love feta. It adds about 30 calories per serving.

1 Heat the olive oil and butter in a large saucepan. Add the onion and fry it for several minutes until it's soft and translucent. Add the garlic, coriander, turmeric and ginger, and then stir for a minute.

2 Add the carrots and celeriac and stir until they're well coated with the spices, then pour in the stock or water and season with salt and pepper. Bring the soup to the boil, then turn the heat down to medium and leave it to simmer for about 15 minutes until the vegetables are nice and tender.

3 Allow the soup to cool slightly, then blitz it in a blender or with a stick blender until smooth. Reheat if necessary, then serve garnished with herbs and feta, if using.

Serves 4

1 tsp olive oil
10g butter
1 large onion, finely chopped
1 garlic clove, finely chopped
1 tbsp ground coriander
pinch of ground turmeric
pinch of ground ginger
250g carrots, thinly sliced
250g celeriac, finely diced
1.2 litres chicken or vegetable stock
    or water
salt and black pepper

To serve
small bunch of coriander, finely
    chopped
a few mint leaves, finely chopped
    (optional)
50g feta cheese, crumbled (optional)

125 calories per serving; 155 with extra feta cheese

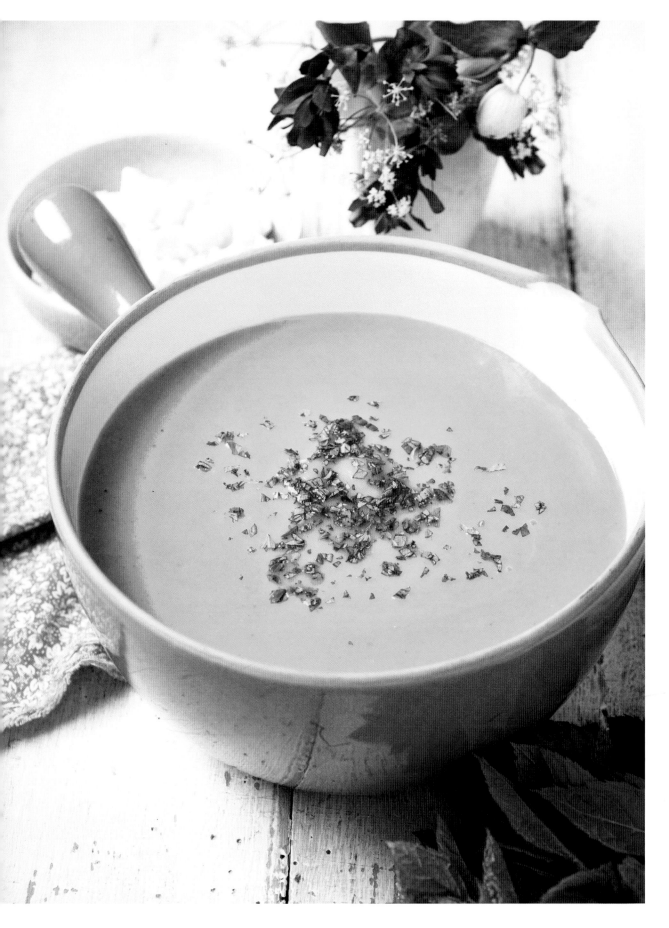

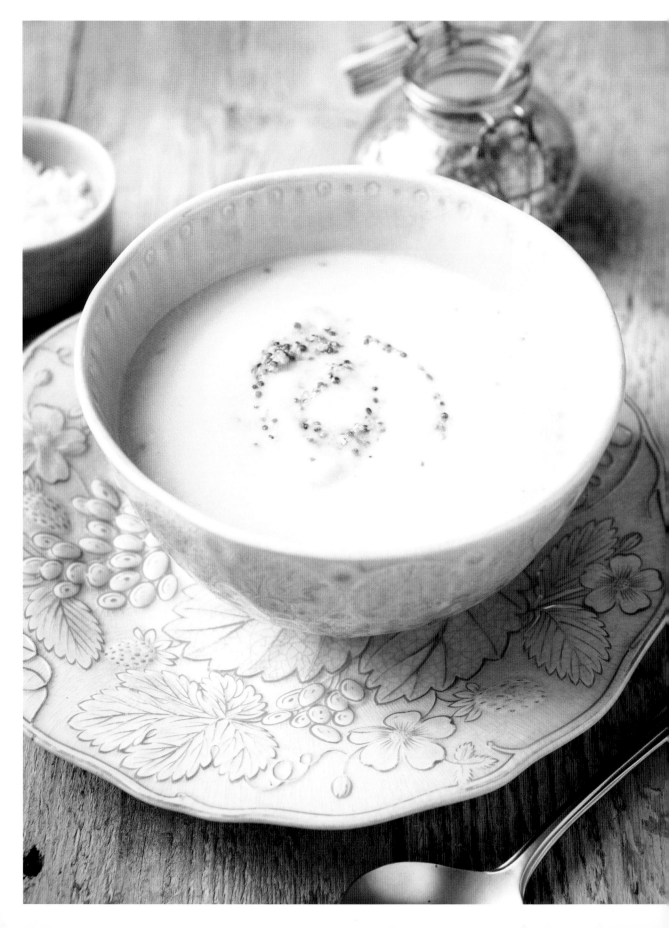

Cauliflower cheese soup

Easier and quicker to make than cauli cheese, this soup still has all that lovely flavour. It's rich, creamy and filling but still reasonably low cal – a great winter warmer. Add a touch of wholegrain mustard before you tuck in.

1 Melt the butter in a large saucepan, then add the onion, garlic and cauliflower florets. Put a lid on the pan and cook the vegetables over a low heat for 5 minutes, stirring every so often. Pour in the stock, then season with salt and white pepper.

2 Simmer the soup, uncovered, for 15 minutes until the cauliflower is tender, then add the grated cheese and stir until it has melted. Allow the soup to cool slightly, then blitz it in a blender or with a stick blender until smooth.

3 Serve the soup piping hot, adding a swirl of mustard – about half a teaspoon – to each serving and a sprinkling of extra cheese, if you like.

Serves 4

10g butter
1 large onion, finely chopped
1 garlic clove, finely chopped
1 large cauliflower (about 800g),
   broken up into florets
1 litre chicken or vegetable stock
75g Cheddar cheese, grated
salt and white pepper

To serve
wholegrain mustard
25g Cheddar cheese, grated
   (optional)

219 calories per serving; 244 with extra cheese

Gazpacho

This is a summer soup – served icy cold and made when tomatoes are cheap, sun-ripened and really tasty. We grow our own and we literally have a tomato mountain so I'm always looking for good ways to use them up! If you want, you can eke out your tomatoes with a carton of passata but don't use all passata or canned tomatoes, as the soup won't taste as good. You'll see that we've suggested quite a wide margin on the amount of vinegar – this is because some tomatoes are much more acidic than others. Also depends on your personal taste. Love the egg garnish. (Have I mentioned that I ♡ eggs. Arghhhh!)

1 Put the tomatoes (and the passata, if using), with the cucumber, red peppers, garlic and basil leaves in a blender. Season with salt and black pepper and blitz until the mixture is as smooth as you can get it.

2 Pour the soup into a sieve over a large bowl, using the back of a ladle to push it through. If you like, tip anything remaining in the sieve back into the blender, add 100ml of water and blitz again. Push this through the sieve too, then discard anything left in the sieve.

3 Taste the gazpacho for seasoning, then stir in the olive oil. Gradually add the sherry vinegar, tasting until the soup has the right amount of acidity for your liking. Add a dash of Tabasco as well if you like. Chill the soup before serving with any or all of the garnishes.

Serves 4 generously

1kg very ripe tomatoes, cored and roughly chopped or 500g very ripe tomatoes and 500g passata
500g cucumber (1 large), peeled and roughly chopped
300g red peppers, deseeded and roughly chopped
2 garlic cloves, chopped
2 tbsp chopped basil leaves
3 tbsp olive oil
2–4 tbsp sherry vinegar
dash of Tabasco sauce (optional)
salt and black pepper

Garnishes
1 egg, hard-boiled, peeled and finely chopped
50g pitted black olives, finely chopped
a few basil leaves, finely chopped
squeeze of lemon juice

213 calories per serving (without garnish)

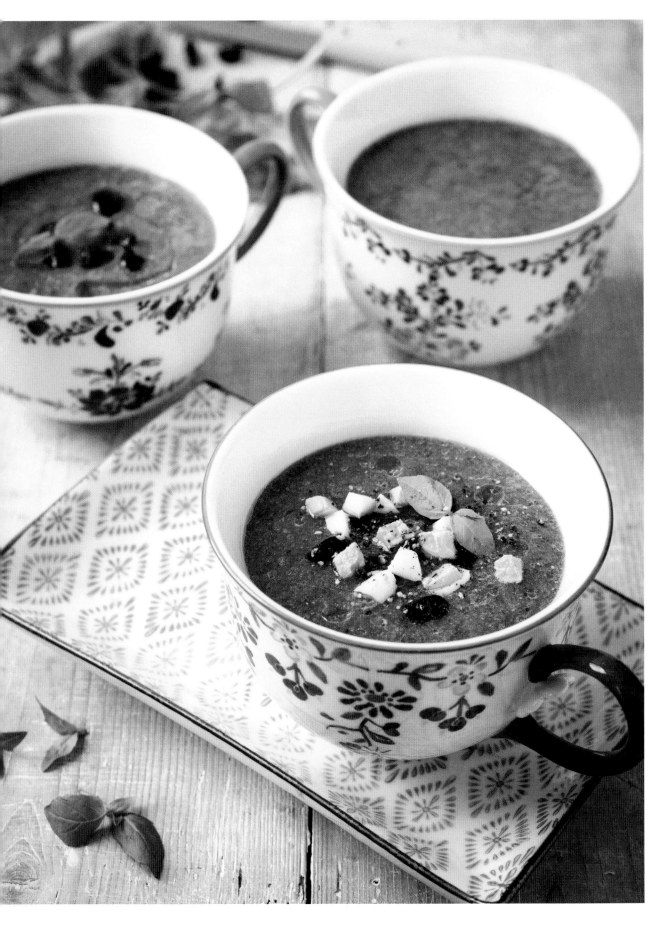

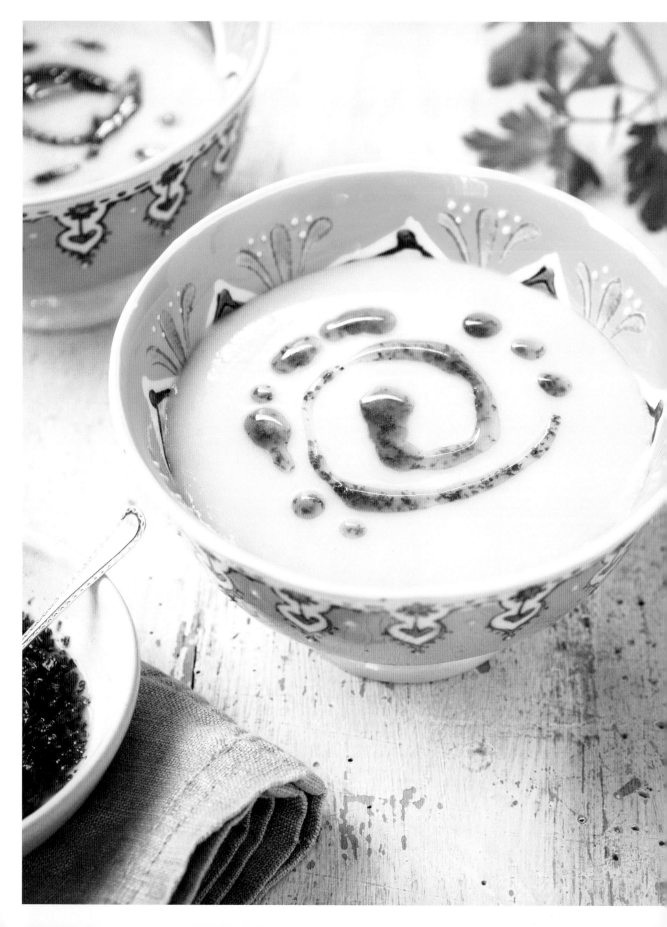

White bean and parsley soup

Dried beans work best for this soup – see page 205 for more info on using pulses. Just remember to soak them the night before. Cooking times do vary, depending on how old the beans are, so keep checking and allow time to cook them for longer if you need to. The parsley oil is amazing.

1 The night before making this soup, put the beans in a large bowl, cover them with plenty of cold water and leave them to soak.

2 The next day, heat the olive oil in a large saucepan. Add the onion, leek and, celery, then fry them very gently for a few minutes until they start to soften. Add the garlic to the pan and cook for another minute.

3 Drain the soaked beans and add them to the saucepan. Pour the stock or water over them and add the parsley and the rosemary, if using. Bring the stock or water to the boil over a high heat and boil the beans for 10 minutes, then reduce the heat and cover the pan. Leave the beans to simmer for up to an hour, checking from 30 minutes onwards to see if they are tender – you want them to be very soft.

4 Remove the sprigs of herbs, let the soup cool slightly, then blitz it in a blender or with a stick blender until smooth. Season with salt and white pepper.

5 To make the oil, put the parsley leaves and the oil in a small food processor, add a pinch of salt and blitz until the oil is flecked with fine parsley. It should be a very bright, vibrant green. Drizzle a little of the oil on to each bowlful of soup.

Serves 4   (F)

300g dried cannellini beans
1 tbsp olive oil
1 onion, finely chopped
1 leek, finely chopped
1 celery stick, finely chopped
2 garlic cloves, finely chopped
1.5 litres chicken or vegetable
    stock or water
sprig of parsley
sprig of rosemary (optional)
salt and white pepper

Parsley oil
4 tbsp finely chopped parsley
    leaves
2 tbsp olive oil

417 calories per serving

Red lentil, squash and tomato soup

Please don't freak out at the list of ingredients – most are spices that you'll probably have around anyway. This is a good-tempered recipe so play around with it if you like and add extras such as diced red pepper (yum). Some chickpea flatbreads (see page 156) on the side are good.

1 Heat the olive oil in a large saucepan and add the onion and butternut squash. Cook them over a fairly low heat until the onion is soft and translucent and the squash has started to soften. Add the garlic, coriander stems, ginger and other spices, then stir to coat the onion and squash.

2 Add the red lentils, then pour the stock into the pan and season with salt and pepper. Bring the stock to the boil, then turn the heat down to medium, put a lid on the pan and cook for 10 minutes. Add the tomatoes and simmer, covered, for another 15–20 minutes.

3 When the lentils have collapsed and everything is tender, you can either blitz the soup to a smooth consistency or leave it with a bit of texture. Sprinkle with the chopped coriander leaves and add a squeeze of lemon juice before serving. If you've included chilli powder, you might like to top each bowlful with a cooling teaspoon of yoghurt.

Serves 4

1 tbsp olive oil
1 large onion, finely chopped
300g butternut squash, diced
2 garlic cloves, finely chopped
small bunch of coriander, stems and leaves separated and finely chopped
½ tsp ground ginger
½ tsp ground turmeric
½ tsp ground cardamom
¼ tsp ground cinnamon
½ tsp chilli powder (optional) or 1 tbsp of your favourite spice blend
150g red lentils, well rinsed
1.2 litres vegetable or chicken stock
400g can of chopped tomatoes
squeeze of lemon juice
4 tsp plain yoghurt (optional)
salt and black pepper

259 calories per serving

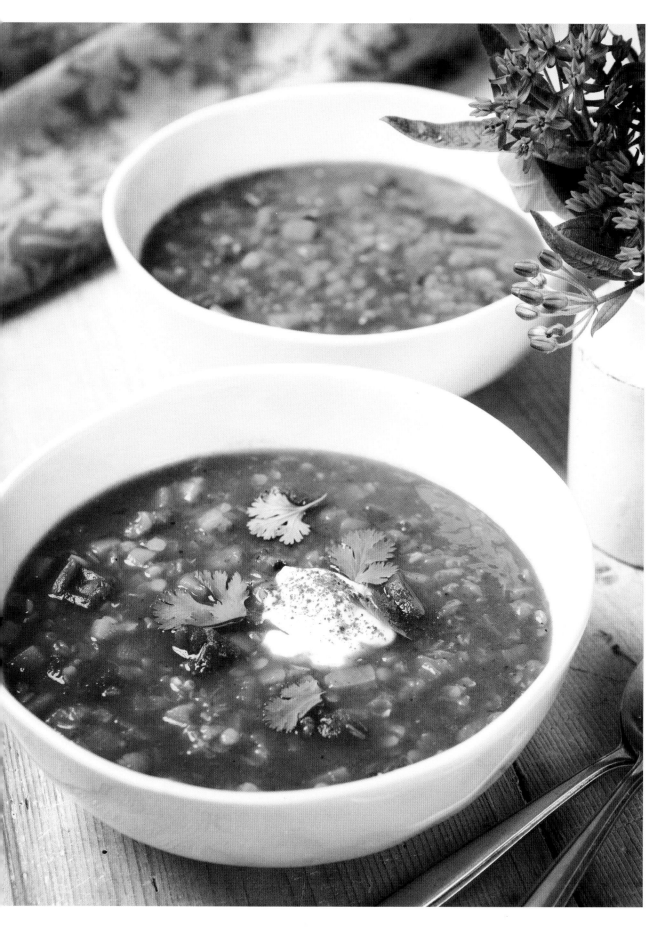

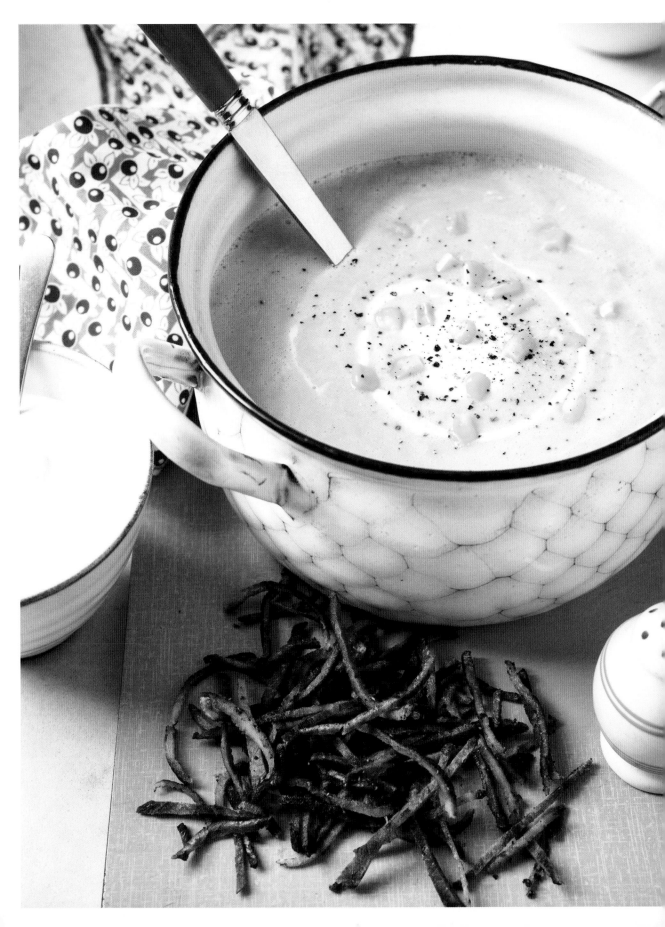

Sweetcorn chowder

OMG this sunny, sweet soup is so quick and easy to make – and it has a yummy bacon garnish. Heat lovers could always add a swirl of chilli sauce too. Yes – I'm talking to you, Matthew.

1 Heat the oil and butter in a large saucepan. When the butter has melted, add the onion and fry it over a gentle heat until it's very soft and translucent. Add the garlic and thyme and stir for a minute, then add the sweetcorn and stock. Season with salt and pepper, then simmer for 5 minutes.

2 Fish out the thyme sprig and remove a tablespoon of sweetcorn to use as a garnish, then blitz the soup until it's well blended. You can make it completely smooth or leave it with a bit of texture – up to you.

3 Dry fry the bacon in a frying pan until it's crisp and brown. Cut the bacon into thin strips or crumble it up into small pieces. Serve the soup garnished with bacon, the reserved sweetcorn kernels and a swirl of crème fraiche.

Serves 4

1 tsp olive oil
10g butter
1 large onion, finely chopped
1 garlic clove, finely chopped
sprig of thyme, left whole
750g sweetcorn (frozen is best), defrosted
1 litre vegetable or chicken stock
salt and black pepper

To serve
4 slices of back bacon
4 tsp crème fraiche

276 calories per serving

REPRO
IMAGE - please lighten the strips of
bacon a little

Thai prawn and coconut soup

I like to get everything prepared for this soup before I start to cook and then I feel like a real pro when I look at all the little bowls. Once that's done the soup is ready in no time. Great with spiralised courgettes if you're into those or with noodles if you're happy with the extra cals.

1 Pour the stock into a saucepan. Add the lemongrass, garlic, lime leaves or zest and the chillies, if using. Season with salt. Bring to the boil, then turn the heat down to a simmer and cover. Simmer the stock for 10 minutes, then strain it through a sieve over a bowl, discarding all the aromatics and reserving the liquid.

2 Pour the stock back into the saucepan and add the coconut milk, fish sauce and lime juice. Simmer for a couple of minutes just to let the flavours combine, then add the baby corn and the sugarsnap peas or mangetout. Simmer gently for 5 minutes.

3 Add the bean sprouts and the prawns and cook for a further minute. Taste for seasoning and add more salt or fish sauce if necessary.

4 If serving the soup with noodles, cook them according to the packet instructions. If serving it with spiralised courgettes, add them to a pan of boiling water and blanch them for 20 seconds, then drain.

5 Ladle the soup into bowls over the noodles or courgettes, then add a sprinkling of chillies and coriander leaves and serve with wedges of lime on the side.

Serves 4

250ml fish, chicken or vegetable stock
2 lemongrass stalks, roughly chopped (no need to remove outer stalks)
3 garlic cloves, thinly sliced
3 kaffir lime leaves or zest of 1 lime
2 red chillies, thinly sliced (optional)
400ml can of coconut milk
2 tbsp fish sauce (nam pla)
juice of 1 lime
100g baby corn
100g sugarsnap peas or mangetout
50g bean sprouts
200g peeled raw prawns
salt

To serve
100g wholegrain soba noodles or 400g courgettes, spiralised
1–2 red chillies, deseeded and finely sliced
coriander leaves
lime wedges

331 calories per serving with noodles; 278 with spiralised courgettes

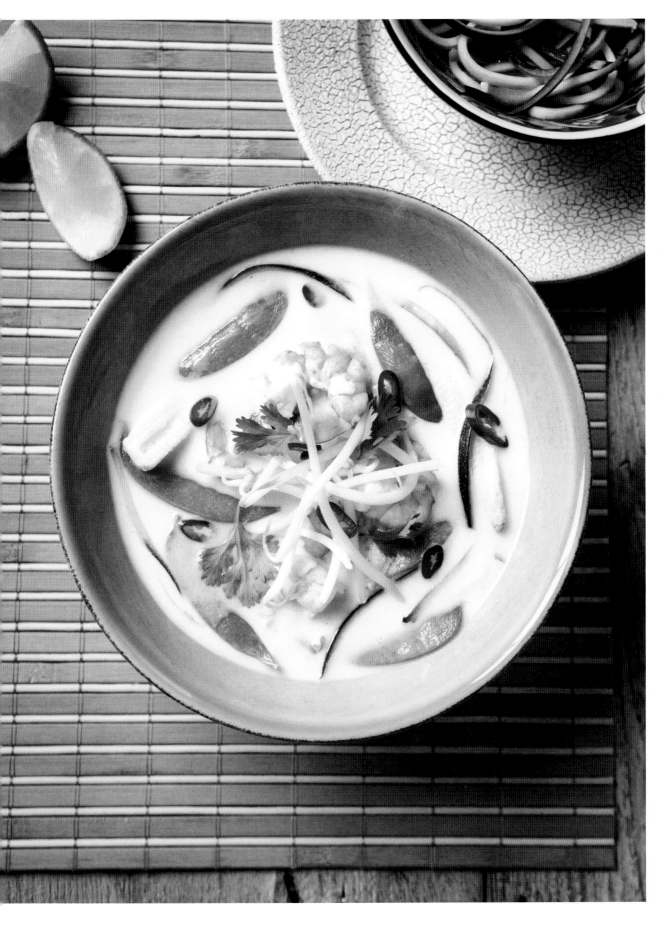

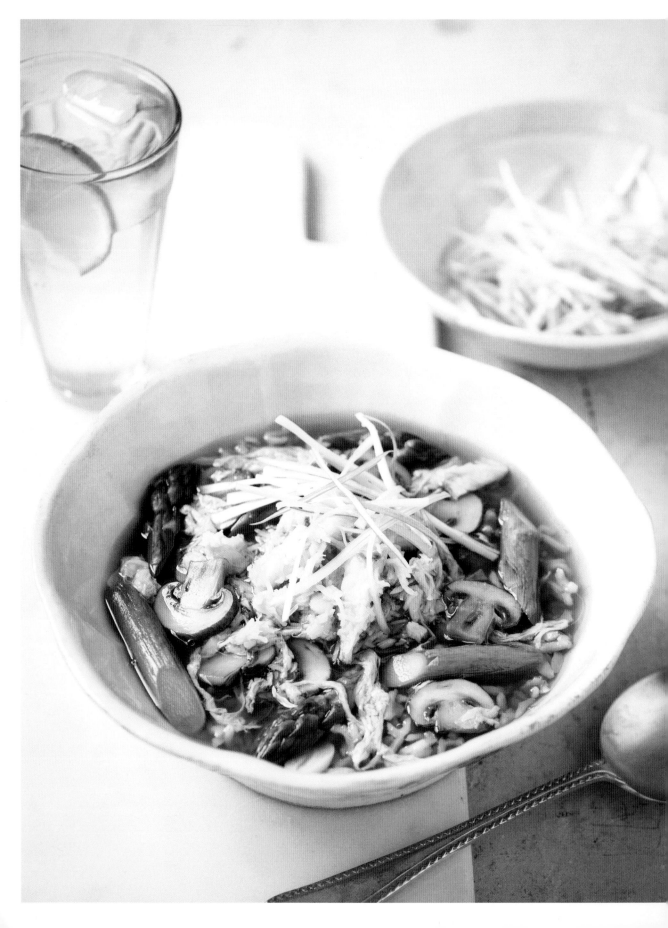

Asian crab and asparagus soup

If you've got some cooked brown rice to hand and all the ingredients prepared, you can have this soup on the table in under 15 minutes. If you don't like crab, just leave it out – the soup will still taste good.

1 If you don't have any leftover brown rice, cook the rice according to the packet instructions.

2 Pour the stock into a large saucepan. Season it with salt, then add the garlic and ginger. Bring the stock to the boil, then turn the heat down and simmer for 5 minutes to allow the flavours of the garlic and ginger to infuse with the stock.

3 Add the asparagus and mushrooms to the pan, then simmer for another 5 minutes. Add the soy sauce, then taste, adding a little more if you think you need it. Pour the egg into the soup, while stirring constantly. The egg will cook instantly, forming long threads.

4 Divide the cooked rice between 4 bowls, then serve the soup immediately, pouring it over the rice. Add a few drops of sesame oil, if using, and a spoonful of the crab meat per serving, then garnish with a sprinkling of spring onions and a few coriander leaves.

Serves 4

165g cooked brown rice
  (50g dry weight)
1 litre chicken or vegetable stock
2 garlic cloves, finely sliced
5g piece of fresh root ginger,
  peeled and finely chopped
250g asparagus, trimmed and
  cut into 4cm lengths
150g mushrooms, left whole
  if small, or sliced
1 tbsp dark soy sauce
1 egg, well beaten
salt

To serve
a few drops of sesame oil
  (optional)
100g white crab meat
4 spring onions, shredded
small bunch of coriander,
  leaves only

171 calories per serving

Summer chicken broth

This has become one of my favourite soups. It's packed with lovely vegetables, is easy to make and everyone enjoys it.

1 Dice the chicken thighs into 1.5cm cubes. Heat the olive oil in a large saucepan. Add the cubes of chicken and fry them briskly on all sides – you might need to do this in batches so you don't overcrowd the pan. As each batch of chicken is browned, remove it with a slotted spoon and set it aside on a plate.

2 Add the butter to the pan. When it has melted, add the onion, fennel and about 2 tablespoons of water. Turn the heat down to low, then put a lid on the pan and cook the vegetables for about 5 minutes until softened. Uncover the pan, add the garlic and stir for a minute.

3 Put the chicken back in the saucepan. Add the courgettes, asparagus and leeks and stir to cover them with the buttery juices. Pour the stock into the pan, add the tarragon and season with salt and pepper.

4 Cover the pan again and leave the soup to simmer over a medium heat for about 10 minutes, until the vegetables are just tender and the chicken is completely cooked through.

5 Mix the cherry tomatoes, basil and olive oil together and season with salt and pepper. Serve the soup piping hot, garnished with the cherry tomatoes.

Serves 4

400g boneless, skinless chicken
   thighs, trimmed of fat
1 tbsp olive oil
5g butter
1 large onion, finely chopped
1 fennel bulb, trimmed and sliced
1 garlic clove, finely chopped
200g courgettes, diced
200g asparagus, trimmed and cut
   into sections
200g leeks, cut into rounds on
   the diagonal
1 litre chicken or vegetable stock
2 large tarragon sprigs, left whole
salt and black pepper

To serve
75g cherry tomatoes, finely diced
small bunch of basil, shredded
1 tsp olive oil

255 calories per serving

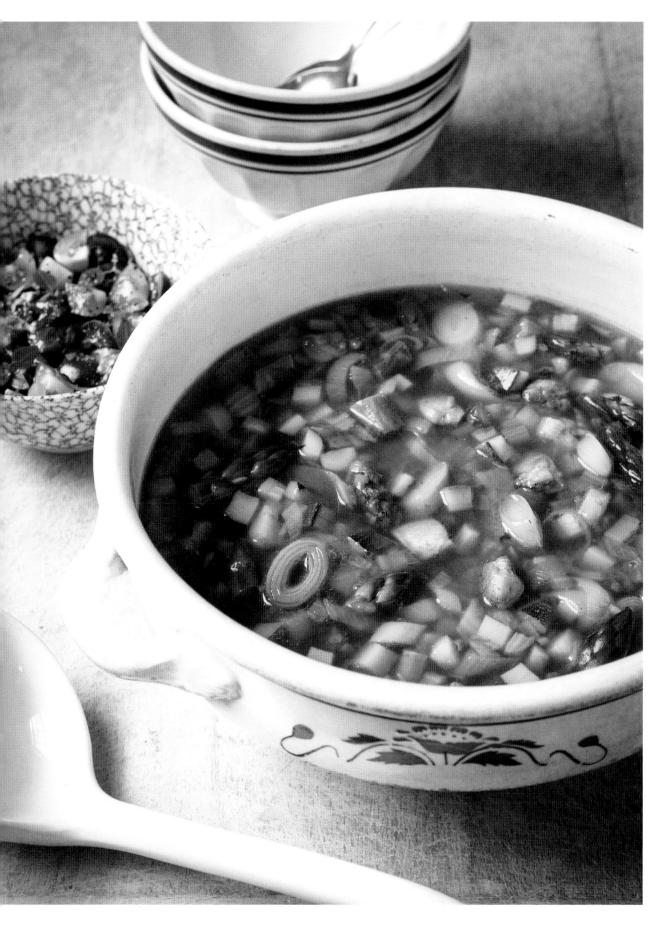

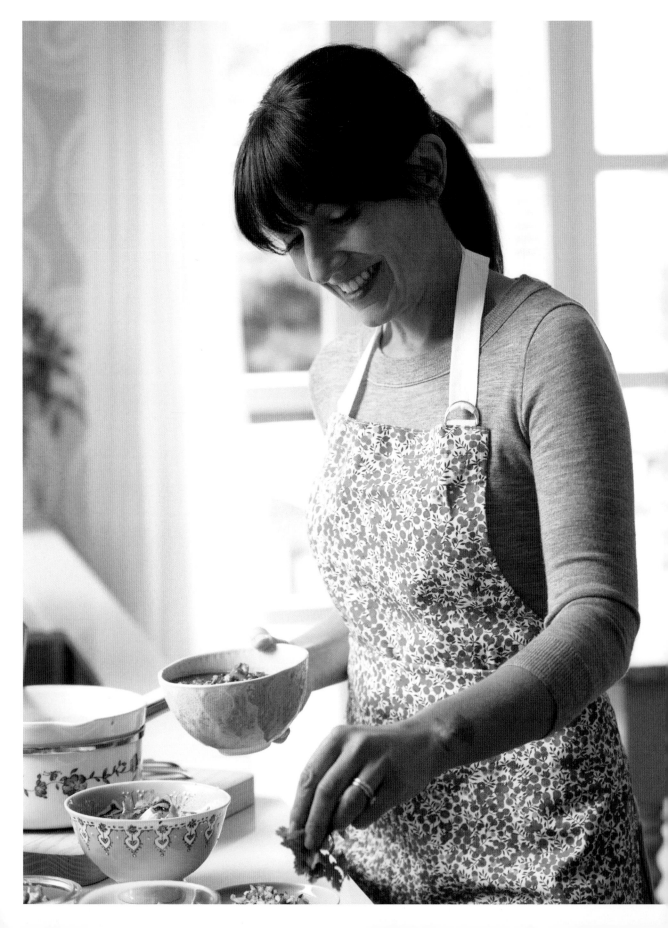

Tex-Mex chicken soup

Another family favourite. Quite a spicy soup this one, but you can leave out the chipotle paste if you want a milder flavour. Or, ladle out bowlfuls for those who don't want the heat, then add the chipotle to the rest and simmer for another minute. That way everyone should be happy.

1 Heat the vegetable oil in a large saucepan. Add the red onion, reserving 2 tablespoons for the garnish, and fry it over a medium heat until it's starting to soften. Add the strips of chicken and sear them on all sides, then turn down the heat and add the chopped garlic. Stir for a minute or so, then stir in the chipotle paste, if using, the cumin, dried oregano and coriander stems.

2 Pour in the chicken stock and the tomatoes, then add the sweet potatoes, black beans and sweetcorn. Season with salt and pepper. Bring the soup to the boil, then simmer for 15 minutes until everything is cooked and the flavours have blended.

3 Mix together the avocado, lime zest and juice, chopped coriander leaves and the reserved onion in a bowl, and season well with salt and pepper. Serve this garnish with the soup so everyone can help themselves and add some lime wedges to squeeze over the top.

Serves 4

1 tbsp vegetable oil
1 large red onion, chopped
4 skinless chicken thigh fillets, cut into thin strips
3 garlic cloves, finely chopped
2 tsp chipotle paste (optional)
2 tsp ground cumin
1 tsp dried oregano
small bunch of coriander, stems and leaves separated, finely chopped
800ml chicken stock
400g can of chopped tomatoes
200g sweet potatoes, diced
400g can of black beans, drained and rinsed
100g sweetcorn (frozen is best), defrosted
salt and black pepper

To serve
1 avocado, flesh finely diced
zest and juice of 1 lime
lime wedges

394 calories per serving

Lamb and barley soup

This is a good meaty soup and a lovely winter warmer but it's still very fresh, thanks to all the greens and herbs. You could use dried rosemary instead of the oregano if you fancy.

1 Heat the olive oil in a large saucepan and add the cubes of lamb. Cook them over a high heat, stirring regularly, until they're seared on all sides. Remove the lamb from the pan and set it aside, then add the onion, carrots and celeriac.

2 Turn the heat down to medium and fry the vegetables for 5 minutes until they're starting to brown around the edges. Put the lamb back in the pan, then sprinkle over the barley and oregano.

3 Whisk the tomato purée into a little of the stock, then pour this over the contents of the pan. Add the remaining stock and season with salt and pepper. Bring to the boil, then cover the pan and turn down the heat. Simmer the soup for 45 minutes, then add the leeks and spring greens. Simmer for another 10–15 minutes until everything is tender.

4 Add the mint or parsley leaves and the lemon juice just before serving the soup.

Serves 4

1 tbsp olive oil
400g lean lamb leg meat, trimmed of fat and cut into 1.5cm cubes
1 large onion, finely chopped
200g carrots, diced
200g celeriac, diced
50g barley
1 tsp dried oregano
1 tbsp tomato purée
1 litre chicken, lamb or vegetable stock
2 leeks, cleaned and cut into rounds
250g spring greens, washed and shredded
salt and black pepper

To serve
finely chopped mint or parsley
juice of ½ lemon

357 calories per serving

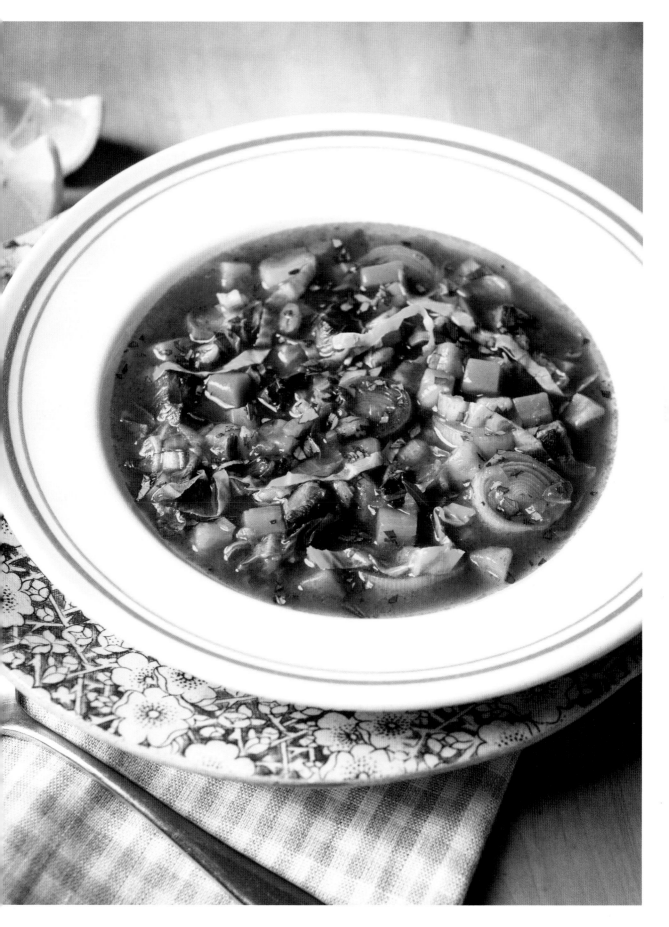

My Faves

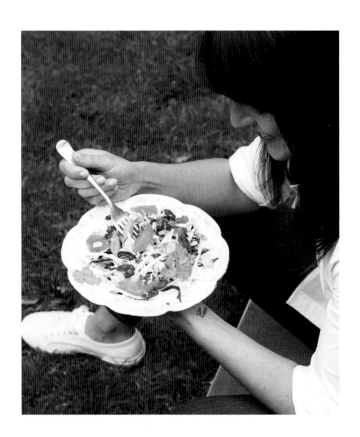

Chapter 3

Salads

"Lots of lovely veggies, a hit of
protein – to keep you fuller for longer –
and all of those satisfying smart carbs.
My perfect meal."

Couscous, orange and goat's cheese salad

You can make this yummy salad with any kind of couscous, but I've really taken to barley couscous lately. It's made from barley, obvs, so is great for anyone who's wheat-intolerant. And it tastes great.

1 Cook the couscous according to the packet instructions and leave it to stand while you prepare the other ingredients. Put the pine nuts in a dry frying pan and place the pan over a medium heat. Toast the pine nuts gently until they're lightly browned, shaking the pan regularly so they don't burn, then set them aside.

2 Prepare the oranges. Slice off the tops and bottoms, then stand one of the oranges upright on a chopping board. Following the curve of the fruit, slice off the skin from top to bottom, then trim off any remaining pith. Hold the orange in your hand and cut out the orange segments as close to the membrane as you can – do this over a bowl to catch any juice. Reserve the juice and the pieces of membrane. Repeat with the other orange.

3 Arrange the watercress, salad leaves and most of the mint and thyme on a large serving platter or on individual plates. Sprinkle over the couscous, then add the orange segments, goat's cheese, olives and pine nuts. Garnish with the remaining mint and thyme leaves.

4 Mix together the olive oil and red wine vinegar in a small bowl and season with salt and pepper. Add the reserved orange juice and squeeze the orange membrane over the bowl to extract any remaining juice. Whisk thoroughly, then pour this dressing over the salad and serve immediately.

Serves 4

150g wholegrain couscous (barley or giant wholegrain couscous also good)
15g pine nuts, lightly toasted
2 oranges
100g watercress
100g salad leaves, such as baby spinach or lamb's lettuce
small bunch of mint, leaves only
a few sprigs of thyme, leaves only
100g rindless goat's cheese, crumbled
75g black olives, pitted

Dressing
1 tbsp olive oil
1 tsp red wine vinegar
salt and black pepper

333 calories per serving

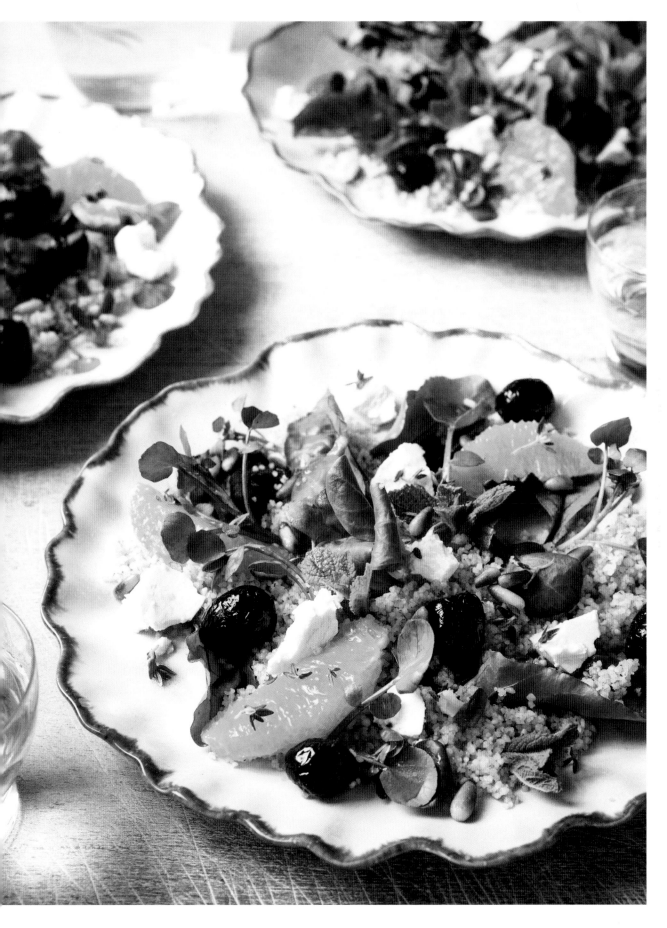

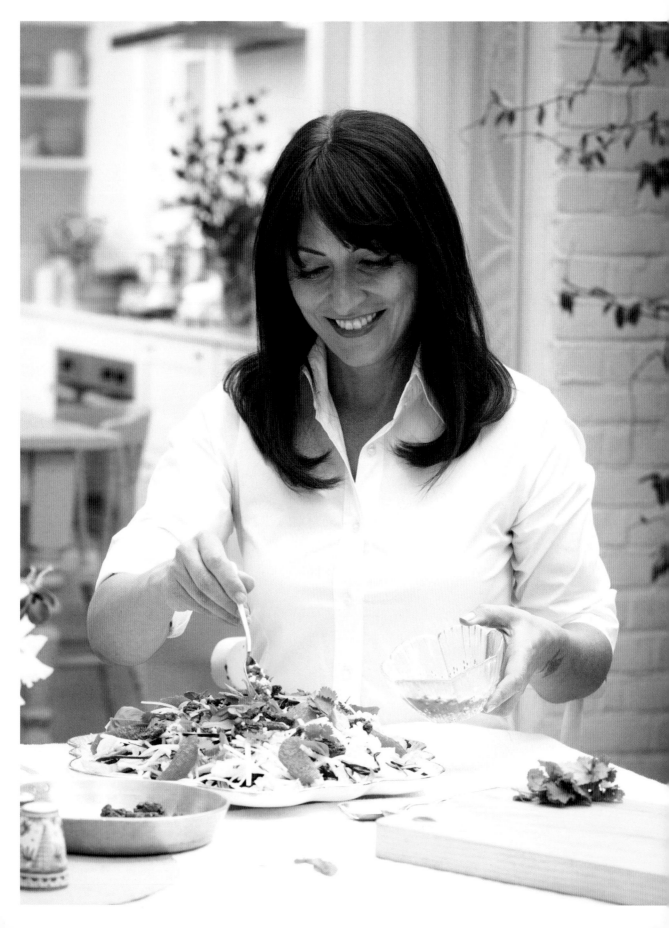

Californian salad

This is based on a salad I ate when I was on holiday in California and loved so much. The original contained Mexican yam, which is hard to find here in England, but we played around with the ingredients and came up with this version. The raw turnip is a real discovery for me. I felt like a Neanderthal when I confessed I thought it would taste like parsnip – actually it tastes like a mellow radish. Who'd 'ave thunk it? Delish.

1 Start by caramelising the pecans. Put them in a dry frying pan and toast them lightly for a couple of minutes, stirring constantly until they start to smell nutty. Add a pinch of salt, then pour the maple syrup over the nuts. Keep stirring the pecans over a medium heat until the liquid from the maple syrup evaporates. It will go sticky for a very short while, but don't panic – carry on stirring and the syrup will soon turn powdery and finely coat the pecans. Remove the pan from the heat and set the pecans aside.

2 Arrange the cabbage, spring onions and turnip on a large platter. Add the grapefruit or orange segments on top, then tear the leaves from the basil and coriander and sprinkle them on the salad, together with the pecans. Season with salt and pepper.

3 Mix together the fish sauce and lime juice, then stir in the chilli and garlic. Leave the dressing to stand for a few minutes, then pour it over the salad and serve immediately.

Serves 4

50g pecan halves
2 tbsp maple syrup
¼ red cabbage, shredded
¼ white or Chinese cabbage, shredded
small bunch of spring onions, shredded
1 turnip, cut into matchsticks
1 red grapefruit or 1 orange, cut into segments (see p.66)
small bunch of basil
small bunch of coriander
salt and black pepper

Dressing
1 tbsp fish sauce (nam pla)
juice of 1 lime
1 chilli, deseeded and finely chopped
1 garlic clove, finely chopped

175 calories per serving

Mushroom, spinach and tomato salad

This is good served while the mushrooms are still warm. The dressing takes seconds and is brilliantly tasty and fragrant – #soeasy.

1 Heat the olive oil in a large saucepan. Add the mushrooms and fry them gently until they're browned but not completely soft. Season the mushrooms with salt and pepper, then add the garlic and cook for another minute. Sprinkle in the parsley and stir to combine, then remove the pan from the heat and set it aside.

2 Toast the pine nuts gently in a small frying pan until lightly browned, shaking the pan regularly so they don't burn. Set them aside.

3 To make the dressing, put the olive oil and basil in a small food processor with the garlic. Season with salt and pepper, then blitz until you have a green-flecked oil. Add a little water to help the mixture along if necessary.

4 Arrange the spinach, tomatoes and the cooked mushrooms on a large plate, then add the Parmesan shavings and the toasted pine nuts. Drizzle the dressing over the salad and add a few drops of balsamic vinegar or lemon juice.

Serves 4

1 tbsp olive oil
250g white or chestnut
  mushrooms, halved
1 garlic clove, finely chopped
2 tbsp finely chopped parsley
25g pine nuts
250g baby leaf spinach, well
  washed and drained
200g cherry tomatoes, halved
25g Parmesan cheese, cut into
  shavings
a few drops of balsamic vinegar
  or lemon juice
salt and black pepper

Dressing
1 tbsp olive oil
small bunch of basil
1 garlic clove, roughly chopped

161 calories per serving

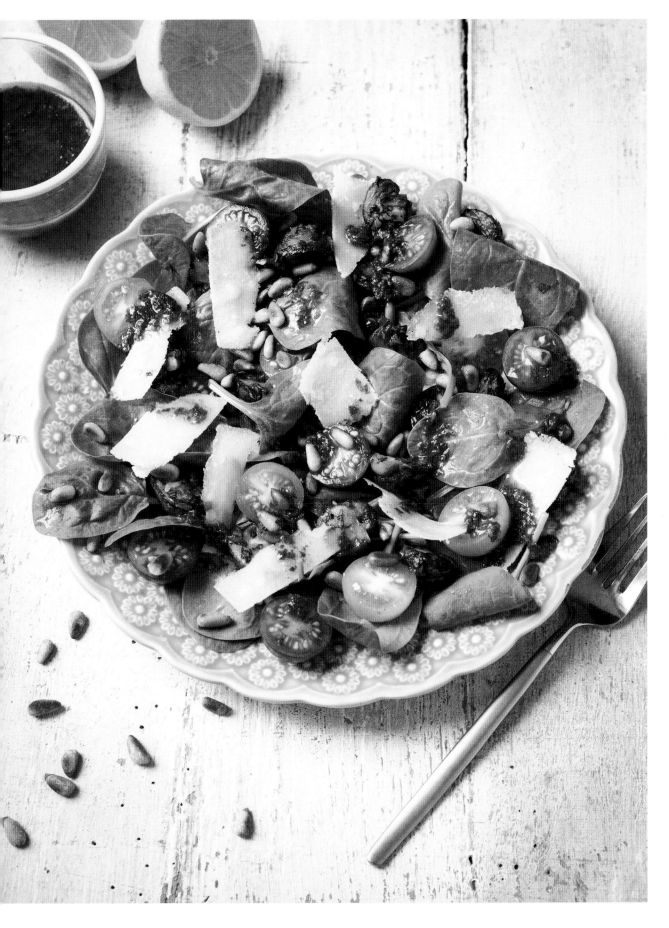

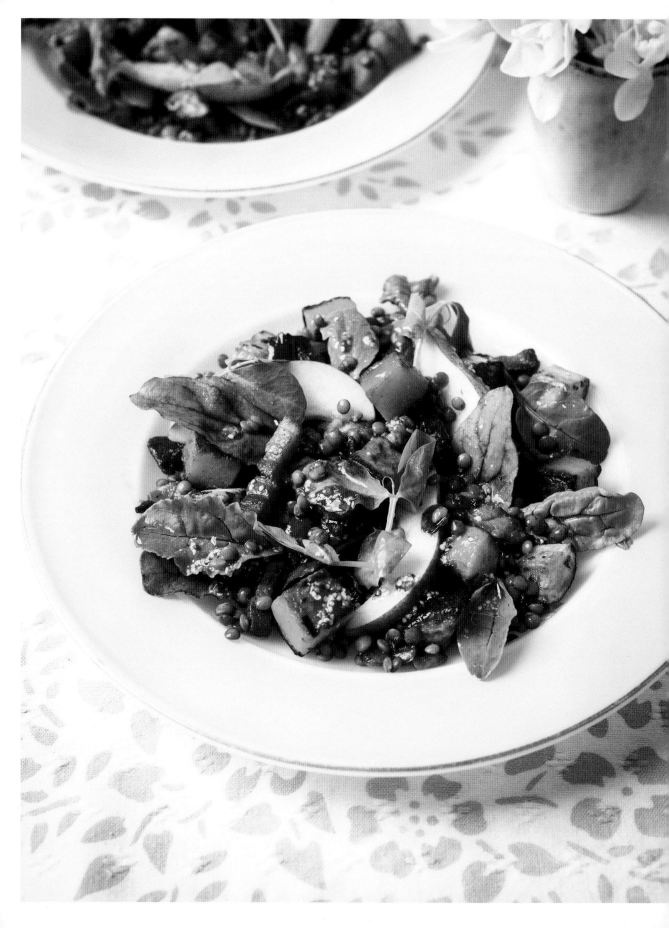

Pumpkin and lentil salad

Lentils are a great smart carb and go beautifully with the soft texture of the pumpkin or squash. A bit of bacon is amazing on this or even some blue cheese if you want to stay veggie – 100 grams of bacon adds about 50 calories per serving; 100 grams of blue cheese adds about 87.

1 Rinse the lentils thoroughly and tip them into a saucepan. Cover them with cold water and bring them to the boil, then simmer for 25–30 minutes until the lentils are cooked but still have a bit of bite to them. Keep an eye on the lentils towards the end of the cooking time, as you don't want them to collapse. Drain the lentils and refresh them under cold running water.

2 Bring a pan of water to the boil, add the cubes of pumpkin or squash and blanch them for 2 minutes. Drain them and set them aside.

3 Heat the oil in a frying pan. Add the bacon, if using, and cook it until some of the fat is starting to ooze out. Add the diced red onion to the pan and cook until it's softened and browning around the edges. Add the pumpkin and courgette, then sprinkle over the sage and season with salt and pepper. Cook the vegetables gently for about 5 minutes until they start to soften and brown, turning them every so often.

4 Arrange the salad leaves on a large plate. Add the cooked lentils, the bacon, if using, then the vegetables and pear slices. Toss very lightly.

5 Whisk the olive oil, vinegar and mustard in a small bowl and thin the mixture with a little water if necessary. Season the dressing with salt and pepper, drizzle it over the salad and serve immediately.

Serves 4

100g green or puy lentils
350g pumpkin or squash, peeled
   and cut into 1.5cm dice
1 tbsp olive or sunflower oil
100g bacon lardons (optional)
1 red onion, diced
300g courgette, diced
1 tsp dried sage
100g salad leaves
2 pears, cored and sliced
salt and black pepper

Dressing
1 tbsp olive oil
1 tsp cider or red wine vinegar
1 tsp mustard

269 calories per serving

Mediterranean roasted vegetable salad

With the feta and bulgur, this salad makes a really satisfying meal. I like to eat it when the veg are still warm and lovely and gooey. Delicious.

1 Preheat the oven to 200°C/180°C Fan/Gas 6. Arrange the peppers, courgettes and onions in a roasting tin. Sprinkle the oregano on top, tuck in the garlic cloves, then drizzle the veg with 1 tablespoon of the olive oil and half the lemon juice.

2 Roast the vegetables in the preheated oven for 30 minutes, turning them in the tin a couple of times to make sure they don't get too brown. Dot the cherry tomatoes and cubes of feta over the veg and bake for another 10 minutes. Remove the vegetables from the oven and allow them to cool a little.

3 Cook the bulgur wheat according to the packet instructions. Allow it to cool, then stir in most of the herbs, reserving a tablespoon of each to add at the end.

4 Squeeze the garlic flesh out of the skins and mash it with the rest of the olive oil and lemon juice and the spices to make the dressing. Season with salt and pepper.

5 Arrange the salad leaves over a large plate and top with the bulgur wheat, roast vegetables and feta. Sprinkle with the remaining herbs and drizzle the dressing over the top.

Serves 4

2 red peppers, (about 300g), deseeded and cut in thick strips
2 medium courgettes (about 400g), sliced on the diagonal
2 red onions, cut into wedges
1 tsp dried oregano
4 garlic cloves, unpeeled
3 tbsp olive oil
juice of 1 lemon
200g cherry plum tomatoes, cut in half
200g feta cheese, cut into cubes
150g bulgur wheat
large bunch of parsley, finely chopped
small bunch of mint finely chopped
1 tsp ground cumin
pinch of cinnamon
pinch of cayenne or chilli powder
100g salad leaves
salt and black pepper

190 calories per serving

Marinated salmon with Asian coleslaw

1 Cut the salmon into 3cm cubes and put them in a bowl. Mix together the soy sauce, ginger, garlic and five-spice in a small jug and pour this mixture over the cubes of salmon. Leave them to marinate for at least 30 minutes, but no longer than 2 hours.

2 Spray a large frying pan with oil and heat until it's very hot. Cook the cubes of salmon for a couple of minutes on each side, leaving them slightly pink in the middle. Set them aside.

3 The easiest way to shred the broccoli is on a mandolin with a shredding setting. Otherwise cut it into very thin slices by hand, then into thin matchsticks.

4 Mix all the vegetables together and arrange them on a large platter, topping them with the coriander, if using. Whisk together all the dressing ingredients. Arrange the salmon over the vegetables, then drizzle with the dressing and sprinkle the sesame seeds on top.

Serves 4

500g salmon fillets, skinned
2 tbsp soy sauce
10g fresh root ginger, grated
2 garlic cloves, finely chopped
½ tsp Chinese five-spice powder
olive oil spray
200g broccoli
200g Chinese white cabbage, shredded
1 courgette, cut into thin strips
100g mooli or radishes, shredded
chopped coriander (optional)
2 tsp black sesame seeds

Dressing
2 tbsp soy sauce
1 tbsp olive or vegetable oil
juice of 1 lime
1 garlic clove, finely chopped

320 calories per serving

Smoked fish and beetroot salad

1 Cut the apple and celeriac into thin matchsticks and put them in a bowl. Mix a teaspoon of the lemon juice with a tablespoon of water and pour it over, mixing well, to stop the apple and celeriac turning brown.

2 Arrange the salad leaves on a large platter or in a bowl. Sprinkle the celeriac and apple on top, followed by the shallot. Remove the skin from the mackerel and pull the flesh into chunks and add them to the salad. Cut the beetroot into wedges and add those too.

3 Whisk the rest of the lemon juice with the oil and mustard and season with salt and pepper. If the dressing seems too thick, thin it with a tablespoon of water, then drizzle it over the salad and serve.

Serves 4

1 eating apple
100g celeriac
juice of 1 lemon
150g salad leaves, well washed
1 shallot, thinly sliced
250g smoked mackerel fillets
400g cooked beetroot
1 tbsp olive oil
1 tsp mustard
salt and black pepper

308 calories per serving

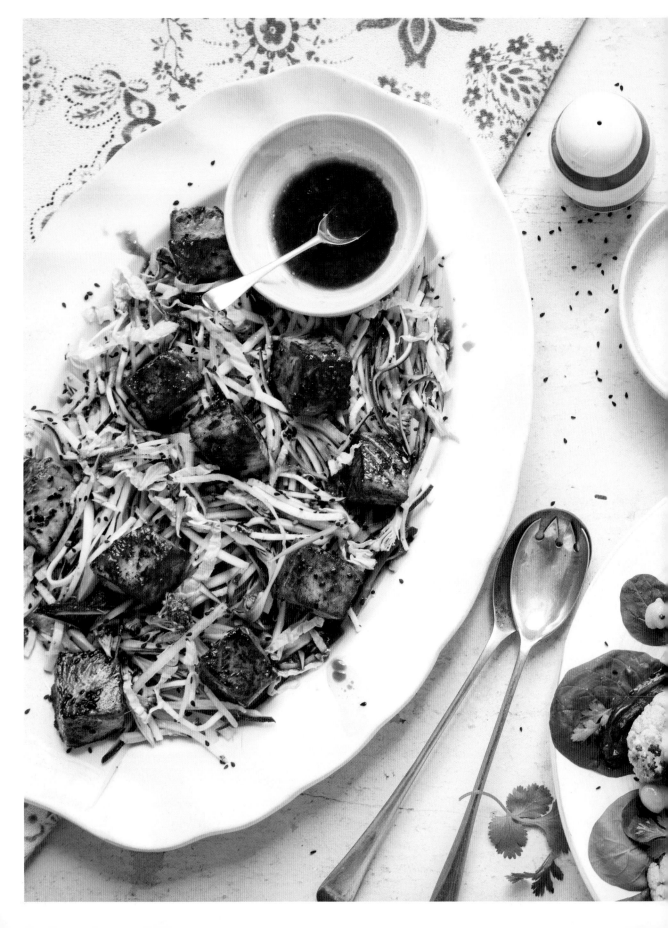

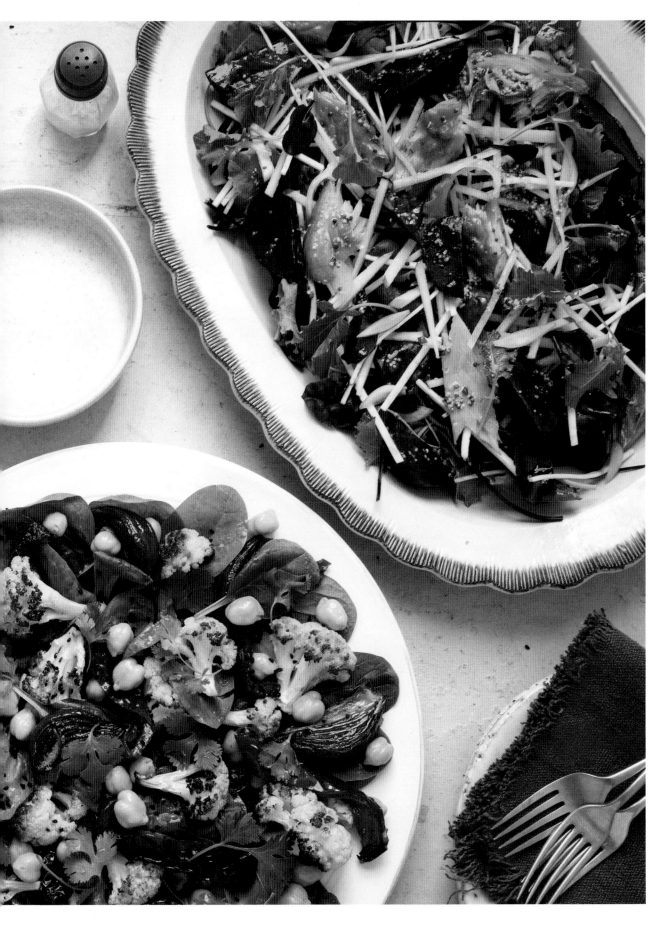

Thai prawn salad

This is a simpler version of that much-loved dish, pad thai, but without the noodles. You can, of course, add noodles for anyone who wants a more substantial salad. In case you're wondering – green papaya is simply unripe papaya and is a popular ingredient in Thai and Vietnamese salads – goes really well with chilli and lime. Tamarind paste has a sweet and sour taste and is available in most supermarkets. If you don't have any, just leave it out – I won't tell anyone.

1 Put the prawns in a bowl and season them with salt and the lime zest, turning them gently so they are all lightly coated. Heat the oil in a frying pan and add the garlic. After a few seconds, add the prawns and cook them on each side until they are pink and opaque. Remove them from the pan and set them aside to cool.

2 Arrange the lettuce or cabbage, cucumber and bean sprouts in a large shallow bowl or on a platter. Sprinkle over the grated papaya, if using, then the carrots and spring onions.

3 Toast the peanuts lightly in a dry frying pan until they turn a light golden brown, then crush them until they're quite fine. Add the prawns to the salad, then garnish with the peanuts and the herbs.

4 Whisk together all the dressing ingredients and season with salt and pepper. Drizzle the dressing over the salad and serve immediately.

Serves 4

200g shelled raw prawns
zest of 1 lime
1 tsp vegetable or coconut oil
1 garlic clove, crushed
100g lettuce or Chinese cabbage, shredded
½ cucumber, sliced into thin ribbons
50g bean sprouts
½ green papaya, peeled and grated (optional)
100g carrots, cut into matchsticks
4 spring onions, shredded
20g peanuts
a few coriander leaves
a few mint leaves
salt

Dressing
1 tsp tamarind paste (optional)
1 tbsp fish sauce (nam pla)
½ tsp honey
juice of 1 lime
2 red chillies, deseeded and finely chopped
salt and black pepper

115 calories per serving

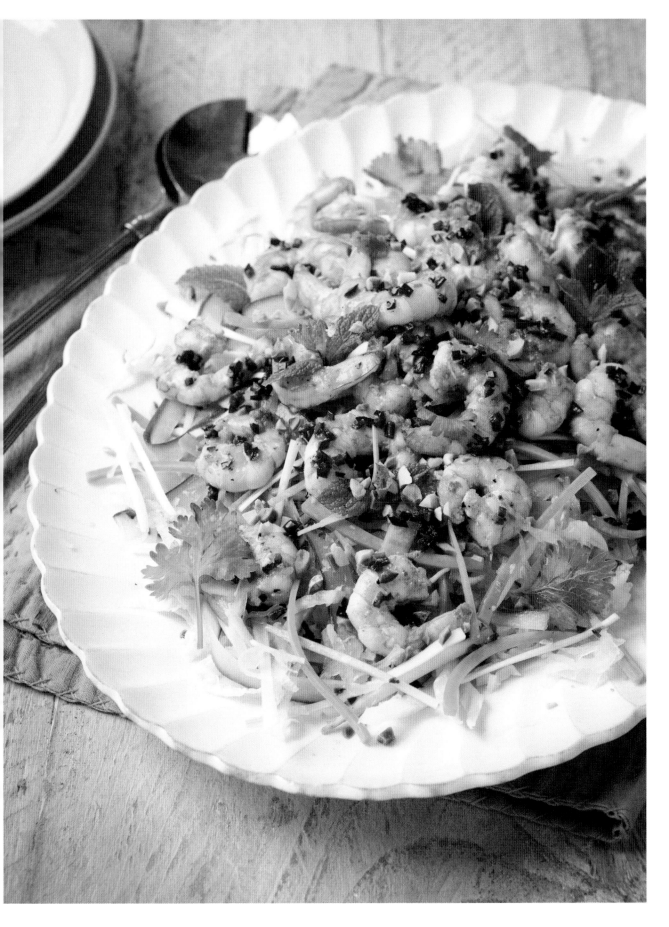

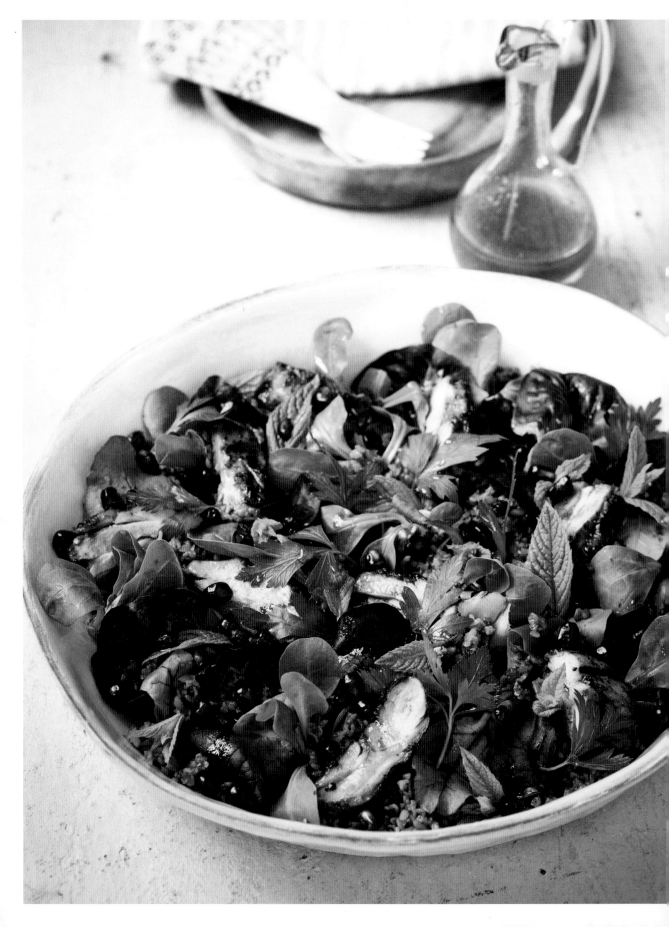

Harissa chicken and freekeh salad

Harissa is a scrumptious spicy paste that's used in lots of North African and Middle Eastern dishes and you can buy it in supermarkets now. Some brands are much hotter than others though, so watch out and taste before you add too much. Some of them also contain sugar – check the ingredients and go for a sugar-free version. Freekeh was a new one on me, but I love it now I've made this salad. It's a bit like bulgur but has a more interesting smoky flavour because the grain is roasted after harvesting.

1 Cut shallow slits in the chicken thighs and put them in a bowl. Whisk together the harissa paste and lemon juice and season with salt and pepper. Pour this mixture over the chicken and turn the thighs over to make sure they are well coated. Leave the chicken to marinate for at least half an hour – or overnight if you wish.

2 When you're ready to make the salad, wash the freekeh and soak it in a bowl of cold water for 5 minutes. Drain the freekeh thoroughly. Heat the olive oil in a medium saucepan, then add the freekeh and garlic. Cook for a couple of minutes to toast the freekeh, then add the stock and allspice and season with salt and pepper. Bring to the boil, then cover the pan and turn down the heat to a low simmer. Cook for 15 minutes, then remove the pan from the heat and leave the freekeh to steam for another 5 minutes. Set it aside to cool to room temperature.

3 Heat a griddle pan until it's very hot. Scrape off any excess marinade from the chicken thighs, then grill them for 5–7 minutes until cooked through and well browned. Remove the chicken thighs from the griddle and cut them into slices.

4 To make the dressing, whisk the oil with the lemon juice and pomegranate molasses in a small jug. Season with salt and pepper and add the garlic.

5 To assemble the salad, arrange the salad leaves on a large platter and spoon over a tablespoon of the dressing. Cover with the freekeh. Arrange the chicken over the freekeh, then sprinkle with the herbs and pomegranate seeds. Drizzle over the rest of the dressing and serve immediately.

Serves 4

400g boneless, skinless chicken thighs, trimmed of fat
2 tbsp harissa paste
juice of 1 lemon
100g freekeh
1 tsp olive oil
2 garlic cloves, finely chopped
200ml chicken or vegetable stock
½ tsp ground allspice
150g mixed salad leaves
small bunch of mint, leaves only
small bunch of parsley, leaves only
seeds from ½ pomegranate
salt and black pepper

Dressing
1 tbsp olive oil
juice of 1 lemon
1 tbsp pomegranate molasses
1 garlic clove, crushed

283 calories per serving

Chicken, broccoli and spelt salad

I discovered spelt when we were working on my first cookbook and I love it. It's a grain, with a great nutty flavour and good firm texture. You can cook it yourself, as below, or you can buy it ready cooked in sachets in the supermarket. Up to you. This salad has an anchovy dressing and I didn't think I liked anchovies but I do like them in this – they add lots of flavour.

1 Heat a griddle pan until it's very hot, and spray it with olive oil spray. Add the chicken thighs and grill them for 5–7 minutes on each side until they're cooked through and golden brown. Remove the thighs from the pan and set them aside to cool, then slice them thickly.

2 If you're not using ready-cooked spelt, put the spelt in a saucepan, add plenty of water to cover and season it with a good pinch of salt. Bring the water to the boil, then turn down the heat and simmer the spelt for 15 minutes or according to the packet instructions until the grains have softened but still have a slight bite to them. Drain and allow the spelt to cool.

3 Cook the sprouting broccoli in boiling water for 3–4 minutes until just tender.

4 To make the dressing, finely chop the anchovies and put them in a small saucepan. Add the garlic, lemon juice and olive oil and whisk together over a low heat until the dressing thickens and emulsifies. Add the chilli flakes, if using.

5 To serve, arrange the mixed leaves on a large platter. Sprinkle over the spelt and drizzle with some of the dressing. Top with the sprouting broccoli, cherry tomatoes and chicken and add the rest of the dressing.

Serves 4

olive oil spray
400g boneless, skinless chicken
    thighs, trimmed of fat
100g uncooked spelt, well rinsed
    or 300g ready-cooked spelt
250g sprouting broccoli, trimmed
100g mixed salad leaves, well
    washed
200g cherry tomatoes, halved
salt

Dressing
1 small can of anchovies in olive
    oil (30g drained weight)
1 garlic clove, finely chopped
juice of 1 lemon
1 tbsp olive oil
½ tsp chilli flakes (optional)

286 calories per serving

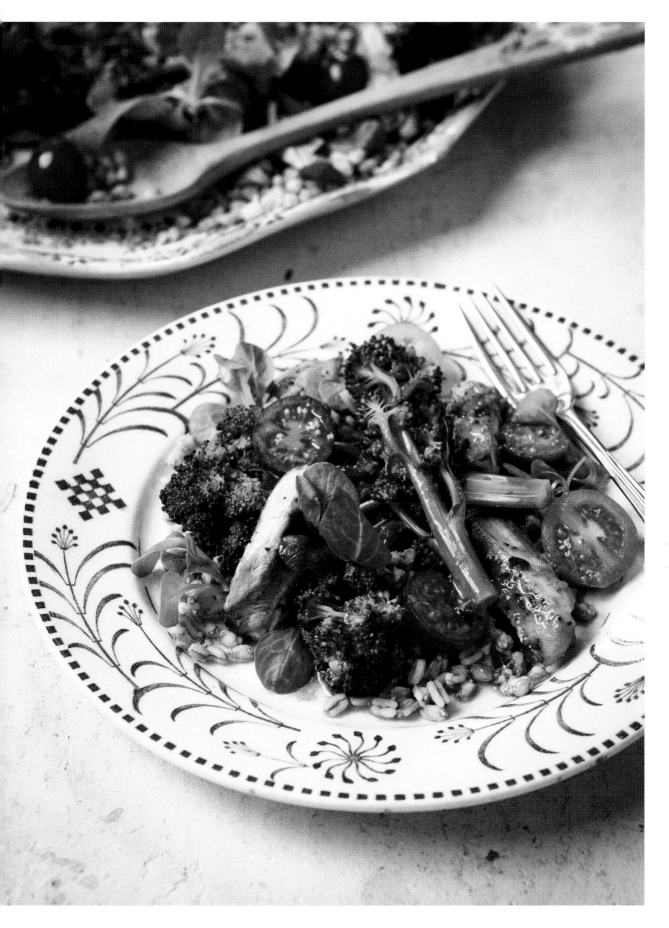

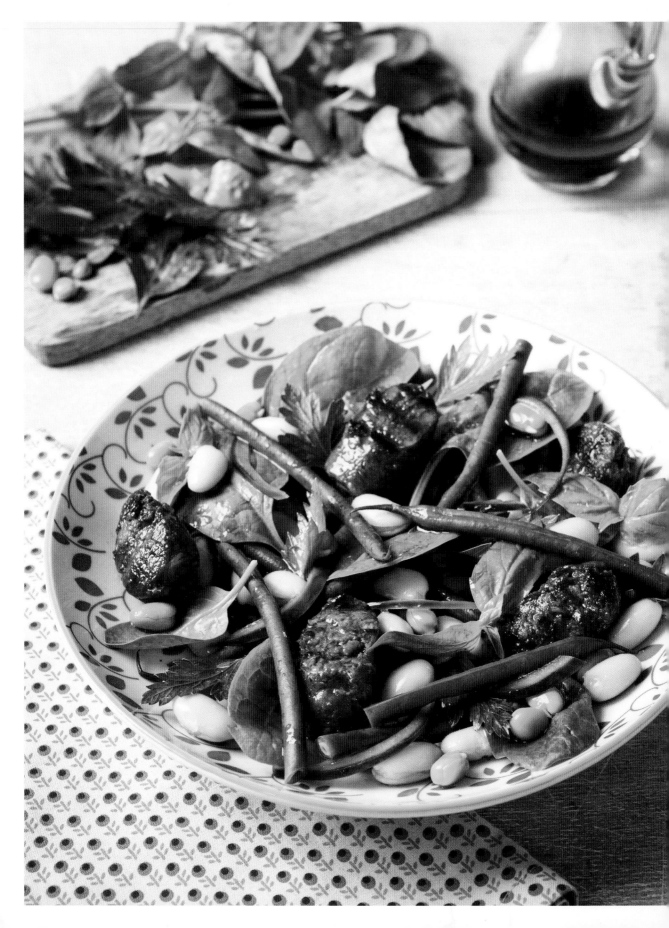

Garlic sausage and bean salad

Sausage and beans but in a salad – keeps everyone happy. This is quick to make too and best served when the sausage and beans are still warm. BTW – I always say chorizo with a sexy Spanish accent.

1 Heat a griddle pan until it's very hot and grill the pieces of sausage for a minute on each side, making sure they have char lines across them. Remove them from the pan and set them aside.

2 Bring a saucepan of salted water to the boil and add the green beans and the broad beans or soya beans. Cook the beans for 3–4 minutes until they're just cooked through, adding the red onion slices for the last minute. Drain the beans and onion slices and set them aside.

3 To make the dressing, whisk the oil and vinegar together in a small jug and season with salt and pepper.

4 Put the spinach in a large salad bowl with the cannellini beans, parsley and basil leaves. Add green and broad beans, onion and sausage and pour over the dressing. Toss the salad well, then serve it immediately.

Serves 4

150g chorizo or garlic sausage, skinned and sliced on the diagonal
250g fine green beans, topped, tails left on
100g broad beans or soya beans (frozen are fine)
½ small red onion, sliced
150g spinach, washed and drained
400g can of cannellini beans, drained and rinsed
small bunch of parsley, chopped
a few basil leaves
salt and black pepper

Dressing
2 tbsp olive oil
1 tbsp red wine or sherry vinegar

276 calories per serving

Beef salad with sundried tomatoes

I learned a good tip with this recipe – soak the shallots before putting them in the salad and they taste good and not sharp at all. Lots of lovely flavours here and you could throw in a few capers too if you like. I don't, but then I'm not a fan. Make sure you take the steaks out of the fridge in plenty of time so they are at room temperature when you cook them.

1 Put the sliced shallots in a small bowl of salted water and leave them to soak for 10 minutes.

2 To make the dressing, put all the ingredients in a small food processor. Blitz until smooth – you may want to thin the dressing with a little water if it's too thick. Season with salt and pepper.

3 Bend each asparagus spear, with more emphasis on the bottom of the stem, until it snaps. This will give you just the tender, non-woody part of the stem. Discard the woody stems. Bring a saucepan of water to the boil, add the asparagus spears and leave them for 1 minute, then drain. Heat a griddle pan until it's very hot. Shake the water from the asparagus and grill the spears for 3–4 minutes, turning them so they get char lines all over. Remove them and cut them into 5cm lengths.

4 Make sure the griddle pan is still very hot. Season the steaks with salt and grill them for 1–2 minutes on each side, depending on how well done you like your meat. Remove the steaks and leave them to rest for at least 5 minutes, then cut them into strips.

5 Arrange the greens on a large serving platter. Drain the shallots and sprinkle them over the greens, together with the parsley. Top with the asparagus and the steak.

6 Drizzle the dressing over the salad and add a few extra strips of sundried tomato if you like, then serve.

Serves 4

2 shallots, thinly sliced
1 bunch of asparagus (about 12 stems, 200g trimmed weight)
600g sirloin or rib-eye steak, trimmed of fat
200g leafy greens such as watercress, rocket, spinach
parsley leaves
salt

Dressing
25g sundried tomatoes, drained, plus a few extra to garnish if you like
2 tbsp olive oil
1 tsp balsamic vinegar
1 garlic clove, finely chopped
2 tbsp roughly chopped basil
2 tbsp roughly chopped parsley
salt and black pepper

322 calories per serving

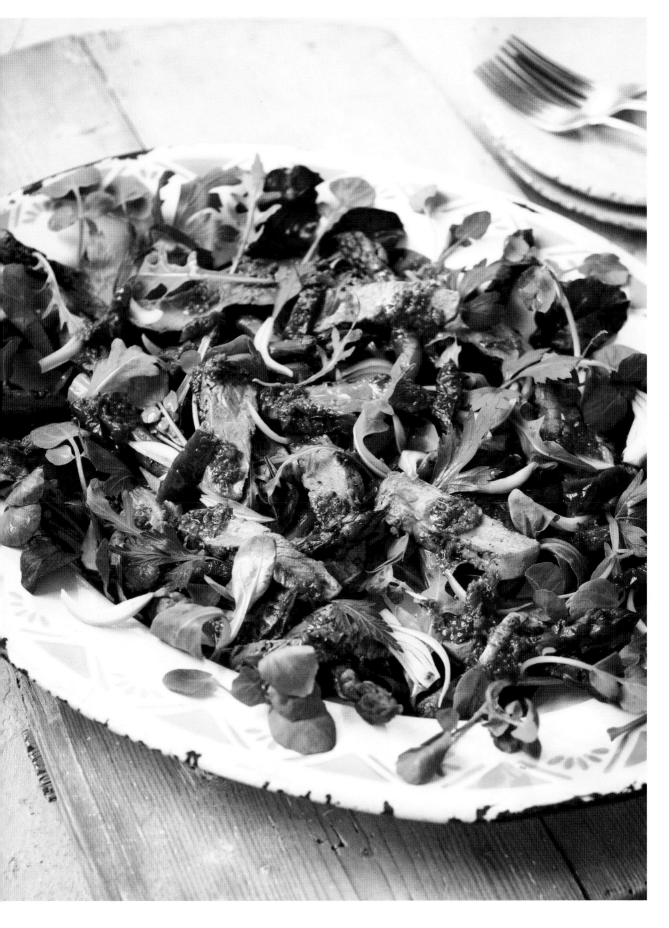

My Faves

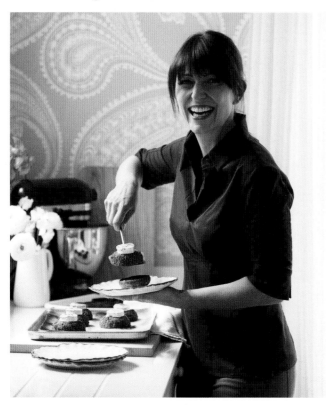

Chapter 4

Veggie + Fish

"You're going to love all these supper dishes. Please try my crazy amazing smart carb lasagne. It's become a regular in my kitchen."

Greek giant beans

This is a luscious side dish but when topped with cubes of feta and served with a salad it also makes a tasty, comforting supper. It's really easy to prepare – just remember to soak the beans overnight – and it freezes well so it's worth making lots and putting some in the freezer for another time. You can do all the cooking on top of the stove if you like, but baking the beans makes them lovely and creamy while still keeping their shape.

1 Put the beans in a large saucepan and add water to cover them generously. Add the parsley and dill stems, bring the water to the boil and cook the beans at a rolling boil for 10 minutes. Turn the heat down, cover the pan and continue to cook the beans for 45 minutes to 1½ hours, checking regularly for doneness. You want the beans to be soft but still with a little bite to them – nowhere near collapsing.

2 While the beans are cooking, heat the olive oil in a large casserole dish. Add the onion, carrots and celery, cover the pan and cook them over a low heat for about 10 minutes or until softened, stirring regularly. Add the garlic and cook for a further minute, then stir in the tomatoes, oregano and the chilli powder or flakes, if using, and season with salt and pepper. Preheat the oven to 180°C/160°C Fan/Gas 4.

3 Drain the butter beans, reserving the cooking liquid. Add the beans to the casserole dish and stir gently to mix them with the rest of the ingredients. Ladle over some of the reserved liquid until the beans are just covered. You will need 200–300ml. Finely chop the parsley and dill leaves and stir them in, then taste for seasoning – the beans will take quite a lot of salt.

4 Put a lid on the casserole dish and place it in the oven for an hour, removing the lid for the last 15 minutes. Add the feta for last 15 minutes of the cooking time.

**Serves 6
(200g portions)**

300g dried butter beans, soaked
   for at least 4 hours
small bunch of parsley, stems
   and leaves separated
large sprig of dill, stems and
   leafy fronds separated
1 tbsp olive oil
1 large onion, finely chopped
2 large carrots, thinly sliced
2 celery sticks, sliced
3 garlic cloves, finely chopped
400g can of chopped tomatoes
1 tsp dried oregano
½ tsp chilli powder or flakes
   (optional)
100g feta cheese, crumbled
salt and pepper

144 calories per serving

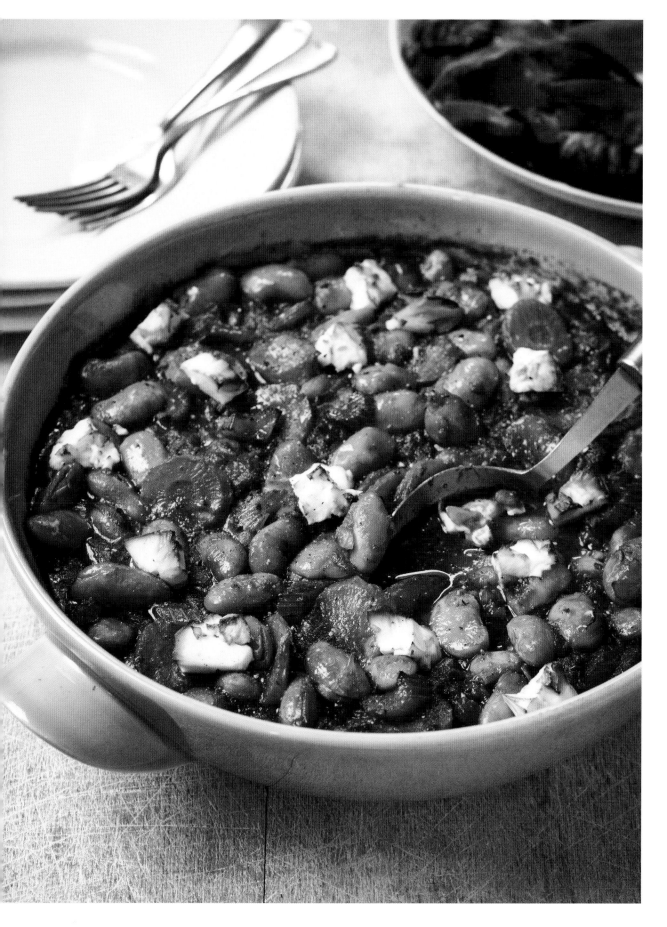

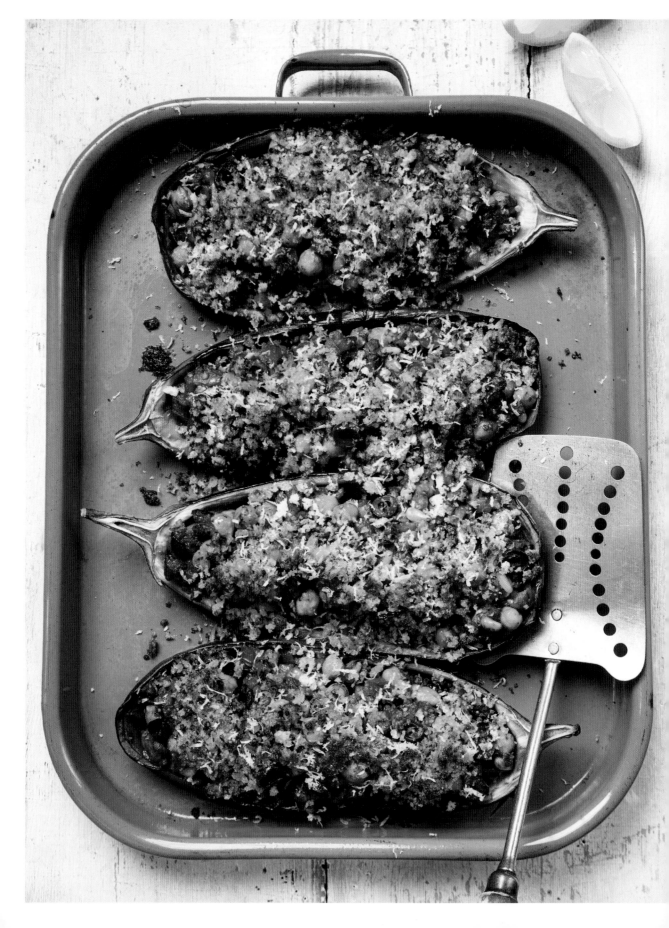

Stuffed aubergines

I haven't always been a fan of stuffed vegetables, but the filling for these aubergines is really tasty and juicy and I love it. The pine nuts are delish, but they do add an extra 40 calories or so to each portion. Add a green salad on the side and that's supper. Big tick for this one.

1 Preheat the oven to 220°C/200°C Fan/Gas 7. Cut the aubergines in half, lengthways, then cut a border, ½–1cm thick, around the cut side of the aubergine and scoop out all the flesh. Dice the cut flesh and set it aside. Spritz the hollowed-out aubergines with spray oil and place them in a roasting tin. Cover them with foil and roast for 20 minutes until they have softened slightly.

2 To make the filling, heat the tablespoon of oil in a wide saucepan. Sauté the onion, pepper and reserved aubergine flesh for a few minutes until they're starting to soften, then add the garlic. Stir for another minute, then add the oregano, half the lemon zest, the chilli flakes, if using, the tomatoes and 100ml of water. Season with salt and pepper.

3 Bring the mixture to the boil, then cover the pan, turn the heat down to a simmer and cook for 10 minutes until the vegetables are tender. Stir in the olives, capers and chickpeas, then half the parsley. Cook, uncovered, for another 5–10 minutes until the sauce has reduced, then stir in the pine nuts, if using.

4 Divide the filling between the aubergine halves – there'll be enough to create a nice domed effect. Mix the Parmesan and breadcrumbs with the remaining parsley and lemon zest, then sprinkle this mixture on top of each aubergine half.

5 Turn the oven down to 200°C/180°C Fan/Gas 6. Put the filled aubergines in the oven and bake them for 15–20 minutes until the filling is piping hot and the tops are browned.

Serves 4

2 large aubergines
olive oil spray
1 tbsp olive oil
1 small onion
½ large red pepper (about 100g)
2 garlic cloves, finely chopped
1 tsp dried oregano
zest of 1 lemon
½ tsp chilli flakes (optional)
200g canned tomatoes
25g black olives, sliced
2 tbsp capers, rinsed
400g can of chickpeas, drained and rinsed or 240–250g cooked chickpeas (see p.205)
4 tbsp finely chopped parsley
25g pine nuts, lightly toasted (optional)
25g Parmesan cheese, grated
25g wholemeal breadcrumbs
salt and black pepper

261 calories per serving

Davina's special lasagne

This is crazy amazing. Using tortilla wraps instead of pasta is such a fabo way of making a lighter than usual lasagne and it's so good to eat. You can also use the chickpea flatbreads (see page 156) instead. Make this in round casserole dish if you have one, so the tortillas fit neatly and you end up with a lovely cake-shaped lasagne that you can cut it into wedges. I like the mozzarella, but you can leave it out to reduce the calories.

1 First make the sauce. Heat the olive oil in a saucepan, then add the onion and red pepper. Cook over a medium heat until the vegetables have softened and the onion is translucent, stirring regularly. Add the garlic and cook for another couple of minutes.

2 Sprinkle over the oregano, then add the tomatoes and season with salt and pepper. Bring the sauce to the boil, then turn down the heat, cover the pan and simmer for 15 minutes. Take the lid off the pan and simmer the sauce for another 10 minutes until it has reduced. Set it aside to cool slightly.

3 To make the filling, wash the spinach well. Don't bother draining it thoroughly, but put it straight into a large saucepan and add the courgette. Cook until the spinach has completely wilted, then drain it in a colander or sieve, squeezing out as much of the water as you can. Leave it to cool, then stir in the ricotta and season with salt and pepper and a grating of nutmeg.

4 Preheat the oven to 200°C/180°C Fan/Gas 6. If possible, use a casserole dish just slightly bigger than your tortillas. Put a quarter of the tomato sauce on the base of the casserole dish and top with a tortilla. Spread the tortilla with a third of the spinach mixture, then top with another tortilla. Add another quarter of sauce, then a tortilla, a layer of spinach and another tortilla, then repeat, finishing with the last of the tomato sauce. Top with the mozzarella, then sprinkle over the grated cheese.

5 Bake the lasagne in the oven for 25–30 minutes until it is brown and bubbling. Serve immediately.

Serves 4–6

Tomato and red pepper sauce
1 tbsp olive oil
1 large onion, finely chopped
1 large red pepper, diced
2 garlic cloves, finely chopped
1 tsp dried oregano
2 x 400g cans of chopped
 tomatoes
salt and black pepper

Spinach and ricotta filling
250g spinach, thick coarse stems
 removed
1 large courgette, grated
250g ricotta
grating of nutmeg

To assemble
6 corn or wholemeal tortilla
 wraps
1 ball of mozzarella, torn
50g hard cheese such as Cheddar
 or Manchego, grated

538 calories per portion
if serving 4; 358 if serving 6

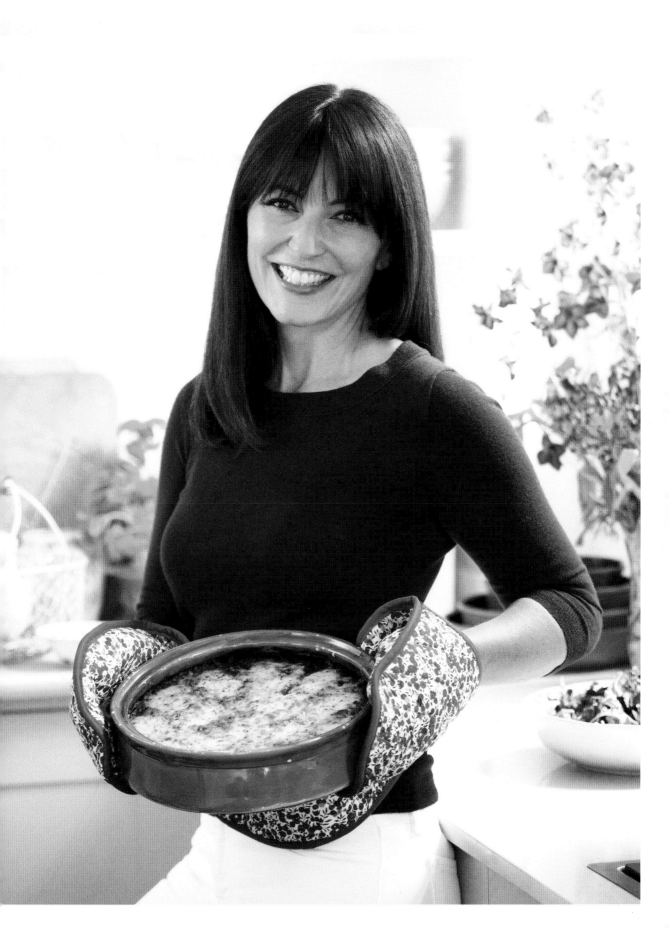

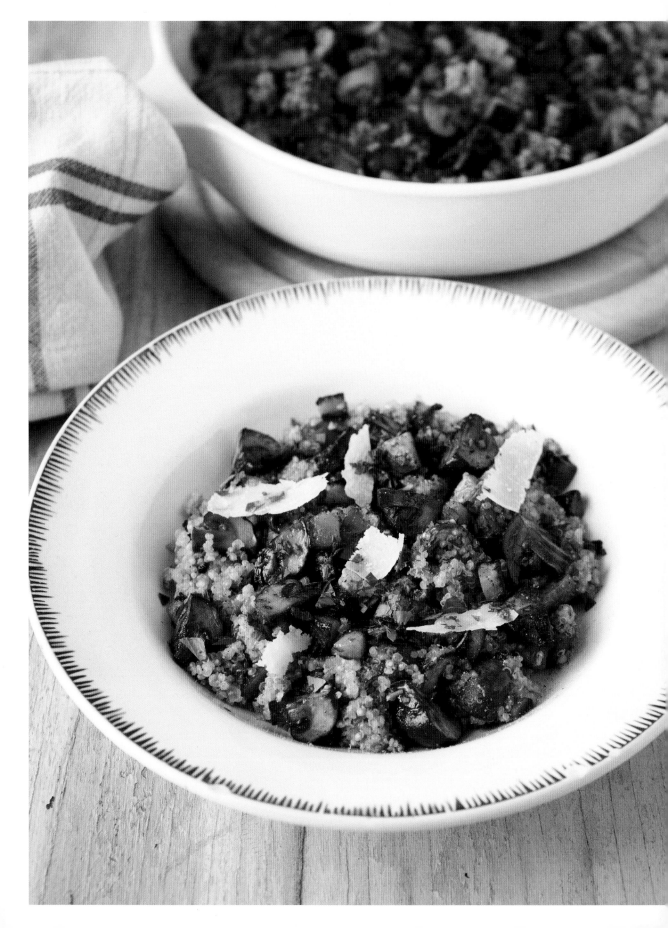

Veggie quinoa risotto

Quinoa makes excellent risotto, but it doesn't release lots of starch like rice does and you don't need to stand and stir it constantly while it cooks. Does make life easier. A good, simple veggie supper.

1 Rinse the quinoa thoroughly, then drain it well. Put the quinoa in a saucepan and toast it over a medium-high heat for a couple of minutes. Pour the stock into the pan, season with salt and bring it to the boil. Cover the pan, turn down the heat and simmer the quinoa for about 15 minutes. Remove the pan from the heat and leave the quinoa to stand, covered, for 5 minutes.

2 Meanwhile, heat the olive oil in a large shallow pan. Add the onion and thyme, and cook it over a gentle heat for 5 minutes, then add the squash and the mushrooms. Cook for another 5 minutes, then add the garlic and allspice. Add 150ml of water, then put a lid on the pan and leave for 5 minutes until the squash is tender.

3 Gently fold the cooked quinoa into the vegetables, then beat in the Parmesan and butter. Serve with a grating of nutmeg and sprinkle the parsley and extra Parmesan on top.

Serves 4

200g quinoa
800ml vegetable stock
1 tbsp olive oil
1 onion, finely chopped
large sprig of thyme, left whole
150g butternut squash, finely chopped
250g mushrooms, finely sliced
2 garlic cloves
½ tsp ground allspice
15g Parmesan cheese, grated
10g butter
salt

To serve
grating of nutmeg
2 tbsp finely chopped parsley
10g Parmesan cheese, grated or cut into shavings

278 calories per serving

Spinach and egg curry

I didn't fancy the idea of this at first, but as soon as I saw a picture of it my mouth started watering and I couldn't wait to get cooking. It's important to use fresh spinach here, as the frozen stuff goes too sludgy.

1 Put a large saucepan over a low heat and add a splash of water to the bottom. Pick over the spinach, removing any very tough stems. Wash the spinach well, without draining it too thoroughly. Gradually add the spinach to the saucepan, pushing it down with a wooden spoon, until it has just wilted – the aim is to keep the lovely fresh green colour.

2 Leave the spinach to drain in a large colander, then squeeze it gently to remove any excess water. Chop the spinach roughly and set it aside.

3 Heat the vegetable or coconut oil in a large saucepan. Add the onion and cook it gently for about 10 minutes until it's soft and translucent, then add the garlic, ginger, coriander stems and curry powder. Cook for another couple of minutes, then pour in the coconut milk and season with salt and pepper.

4 Simmer gently for 10 minutes to let the flavours blend together, then stir in the spinach, along with the lime juice and cumin seeds. Simmer for 5 minutes, adding the peas for the last couple of minutes.

5 Meanwhile, put the eggs in a pan of cold water. Bring the water to the boil and cook the eggs for just 5 minutes so the yolks are still slightly soft. Cool the eggs under cold running water, then peel them very carefully and cut them in half.

6 Put the eggs on top of the curry, then cover the pan and leave the curry to stand while the eggs warm through. Serve garnished with chillies and coriander leaves and some lime wedges on the side.

Serves 4

500g fresh spinach
1 tbsp vegetable or coconut oil
1 large onion, finely sliced
2 garlic cloves, finely chopped
5g fresh root ginger, finely grated
small bunch of coriander, leaves
    and stems separated and finely
    chopped
1 tbsp mild curry powder
400ml coconut milk
juice of ½ lime
½ tsp cumin seeds
200g peas, defrosted
6 eggs
salt and black pepper

Garnish
2 green chillies, deseeded and sliced
reserved coriander leaves
lime wedges

371 calories per serving

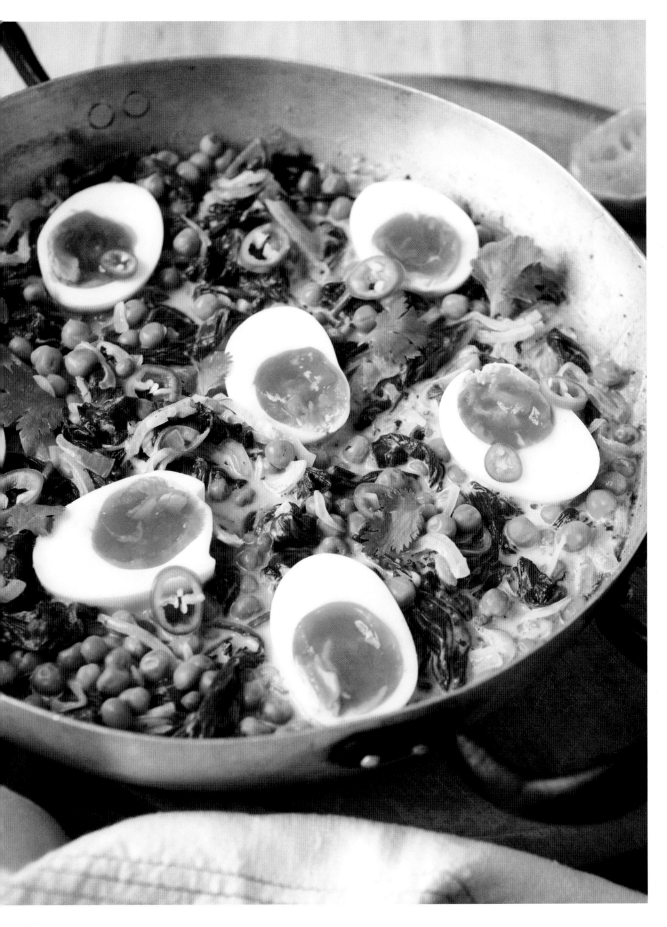

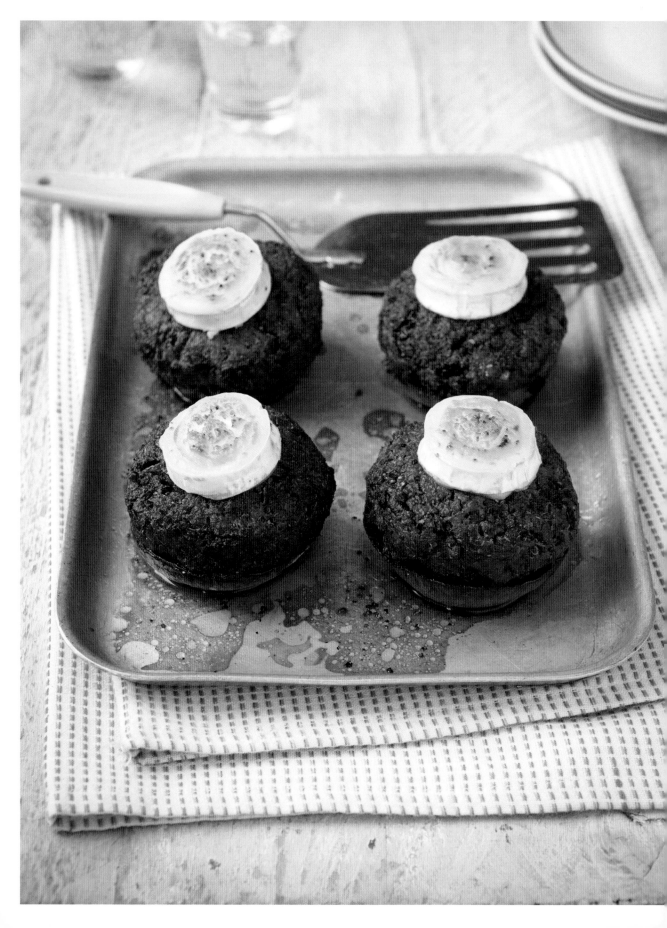

Quinoa and sweet potato burgers

The quantities here are for six large burgers, but they freeze well so if you don't want them all you could stash a couple in the freezer for another time. Lovely served on the mushrooms. BTW, this makes a good vegan meal if you leave out the goat's cheese.

1 Preheat the oven to 200°C/180°C Fan/Gas 6. Using a sharp knife, prick the sweet potatoes quite deeply all over, then put them on a baking tray. Bake the potatoes for about 45 minutes, until they give when you squeeze them. Turn off the oven but leave the sweet potatoes in there to cool – this will help them dry out further.

2 Meanwhile, cook the quinoa. Rinse it thoroughly in cold water, then drain it and put it in a saucepan. Dry fry the quinoa for a few minutes, until it's starting to take on some colour, then pour the stock or water into the pan and season with salt. Bring the liquid to the boil, then turn the heat down to a simmer and cover the pan. Cook the quinoa for 15 minutes or until all the liquid has been absorbed, then remove the pan from the heat. Leave the quinoa to stand for a further 5 minutes.

3 Heat the olive oil in a frying pan and add the red onion. Fry the onion gently until it's soft and translucent, then add the garlic and cook for another couple of minutes. Leave to cool.

4 Preheat the oven again to 200°C/180°C Fan/Gas 6. Remove the skin from the sweet potatoes, then mash them in a bowl with the quinoa and red onion. Add the parsley, paprika and cumin, then season with salt and pepper. Mix thoroughly and form into 6 patties of about 150g each.

5 Place the patties on a baking tray. Trim the stems from the mushrooms and put them on a separate baking tray. Season the mushrooms with salt and pepper, and drizzle them with a little olive oil. Bake the patties and the mushrooms in the oven for 15 minutes, then put the cheese on top of the patties and cook them for another 5 minutes until the cheese has melted.

6 Serve the patties on top of the mushrooms in place of burger buns.

Makes 6 x 150g burgers

500g sweet potatoes
150g quinoa
375ml stock or water
1 tbsp olive oil, plus extra for drizzling
1 red onion, finely chopped
2 garlic cloves, finely chopped
2 tbsp finely chopped parsley
½ tsp sweet smoked paprika
½ tsp ground cumin
6 large field mushrooms
6 slices of goat's cheese
salt and black pepper

330 calories per serving

Paneer and pea curry

This is also excellent made with broad beans. Paneer is a traditional Indian cheese used in cooking and it's fabulous in a curry. It's not expensive and you can buy it in supermarkets. If you don't want to make the spice mix, use a tablespoon of good-quality curry powder instead.

1 First make the spice mix. Put the cinnamon, cumin, cardamom seeds, peppercorns and fennel seeds in a frying pan. Toast them over a medium heat until you can smell their aroma, shaking the pan regularly. Immediately transfer the spices to a plate to cool, then grind them to a fine powder. Mix this with the chilli powder, paprika and ground turmeric.

2 Now for the curry. Heat the vegetable oil in a large saucepan. Fry the onion gently over a low heat until it's soft and translucent, then add the garlic and ginger. Cook for another couple of minutes, then stir in the spice mix and the tomato purée. Continue to cook and stir until the tomato purée starts to separate, then add the tomatoes and 200ml of water. Season with salt and pepper.

3 Simmer for 20 minutes, then remove the pan from the heat and purée the mixture until it's smooth. This is easiest to do with a stick blender, but if you don't have one, use a food processor or blender.

4 Put the pan of curry back on the heat and add the yoghurt. Stir until it's completely combined – don't worry if the sauce looks a bit pale at this stage, as it will darken up as it cooks. Add the paneer and the peas or broad beans.

5 Simmer for 5 minutes, then squeeze over a little lime juice and serve the curry immediately with a sprinkling of coriander leaves.

Serves 4

1 tbsp vegetable oil
1 large onion, finely chopped
2 garlic cloves, finely chopped
10g fresh root ginger, grated
1 tbsp tomato purée
400g can of chopped tomatoes
100ml Greek yoghurt
250g paneer, cut into 1.5cm cubes
100g frozen peas or broad beans, defrosted
squeeze of lime juice
a few coriander leaves, to serve
salt and black pepper

Spice mix
2cm cinnamon stick
1 tsp cumin seeds
6 green cardamom pods, seeds only
1 tsp white peppercorns
1 tsp fennel seeds
½ tsp mild chilli powder
½ tsp sweet paprika
½ tsp ground turmeric

439 calories per serving

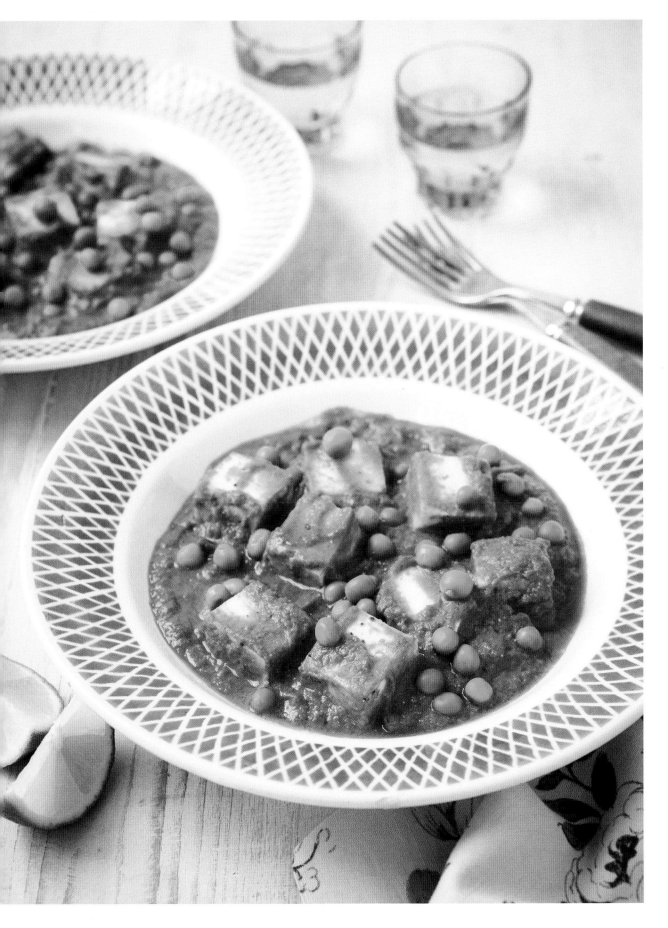

Fresh tomato sauce

Quickest of the quick, this sauce is barely cooked so you get the lovely fresh taste of the tomatoes. Serve with pasta or spiralised courgettes.

1 Heat the olive oil in a frying pan and add the garlic. Cook the garlic for a few moments, then add the tomatoes. Immediately remove the pan from the heat and season the tomatoes with salt and pepper, then leave the sauce to stand while you cook the pasta.

2 Cook the pasta in plenty of boiling water, according to the packet instructions, then drain. If using spiralised courgettes, plunge them into boiling water for 20 seconds, then drain.

3 Pour the contents of the frying pan over the pasta or spiralised courgettes – 'courgetti' and serve immediately, sprinkled with fresh basil leaves and some freshly grated Parmesan, if you like.

Serves 4

2 tbsp olive oil
1 garlic clove, finely chopped
500g ripe fresh tomatoes, chopped
200g wholewheat pasta (or 400g spiralised courgettes)
a handful of fresh basil leaves
grated Parmesan cheese (optional)
salt and black pepper

260 calories per serving with pasta; 105 with spiralised courgettes

Ricotta and herb sauce

Ricotta is an Italian curd cheese and it's available in supermarkets. Just dot it over the pasta and let everyone stir it in for themselves to make a lovely luscious sauce. Long thin pasta such as spaghetti works best here.

1 Whisk the olive oil, lemon juice and zest and mint together in a large bowl and season with salt and pepper.

2 Bring a large saucepan of water to the boil and add a good pinch of salt. Add the pasta and cook for 10 minutes, then add the courgettes and broad beans and cook for a further 2 minutes. By this point the pasta should be nicely cooked but still with a little bite to it (al dente) and the vegetables just cooked through.

3 Strain the pasta and vegetables and add them to the olive oil and lemon juice mixture in the bowl. Divide everything between 4 pasta bowls, then dot spoonfuls of ricotta over each serving.

4 Drizzle with a little more olive oil and sprinkle over the fresh herbs, then serve immediately.

Serves 4

1 tbsp olive oil, plus extra for drizzling
juice and zest of 1 lemon
½ tsp dried mint
200g wholewheat pasta
2 large courgettes, diced
100g broad beans (frozen are fine)
150g fresh ricotta, strained
handful of fresh basil leaves
handful of fresh mint leaves
salt and black pepper

317 calories per serving

Tuna pasta sauce

This makes a great store-cupboard supper. At a pinch you could even do without the onion and garlic if you don't have them, and add some chilli flakes and lemon zest instead.

1 Bring a large saucepan of water to the boil and add salt. Cook the pasta according to the packet instructions. If using spiralised courgettes, add them to a pan of boiling water and cook for 20 seconds.

2 Meanwhile, heat the olive oil in a frying pan. Add the onion and cook until it's soft and translucent, then add the garlic. Cook for a further minute, then add the tuna. Stir to combine everything and add the tomato purée. Keep stirring for a few minutes to make sure the purée is cooked and loses its raw flavour.

3 Add a ladleful (75–100ml) of the pasta cooking water to the sauce. If you aren't serving the sauce with pasta, use hot water or stock instead. Simmer until the sauce has reduced down – it should have quite a creamy texture.

4 Season with salt and pepper, then stir in the olives and capers. Drain the pasta or spiralised courgettes and add them to the pan, then gently mix to coat them with the sauce.

5 Serve with grated Parmesan, if you like, and some basil leaves.

Serves 4

200g wholewheat pasta or
   400g spiralised courgettes
1 tbsp olive oil
1 onion, finely chopped
1 garlic clove, finely chopped
1 small can or jar of tuna, drained
   (about 112g drained weight)
2 tbsp tomato purée
25g black olives, sliced
25g capers
grated Parmesan cheese (optional)
a few basil leaves
salt and black pepper

260 calories per serving with pasta; 105 with spiralised courgettes

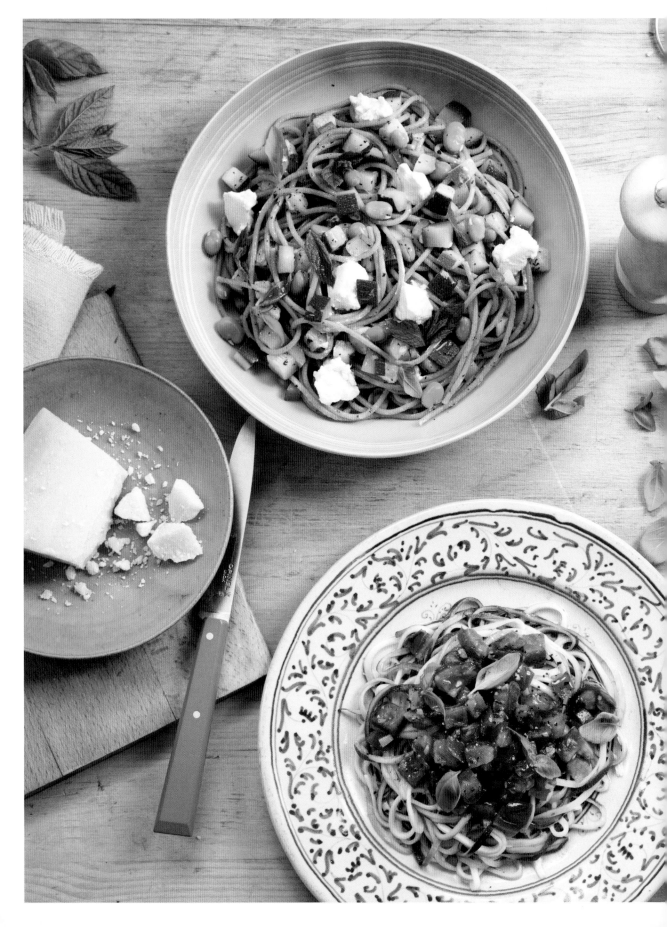

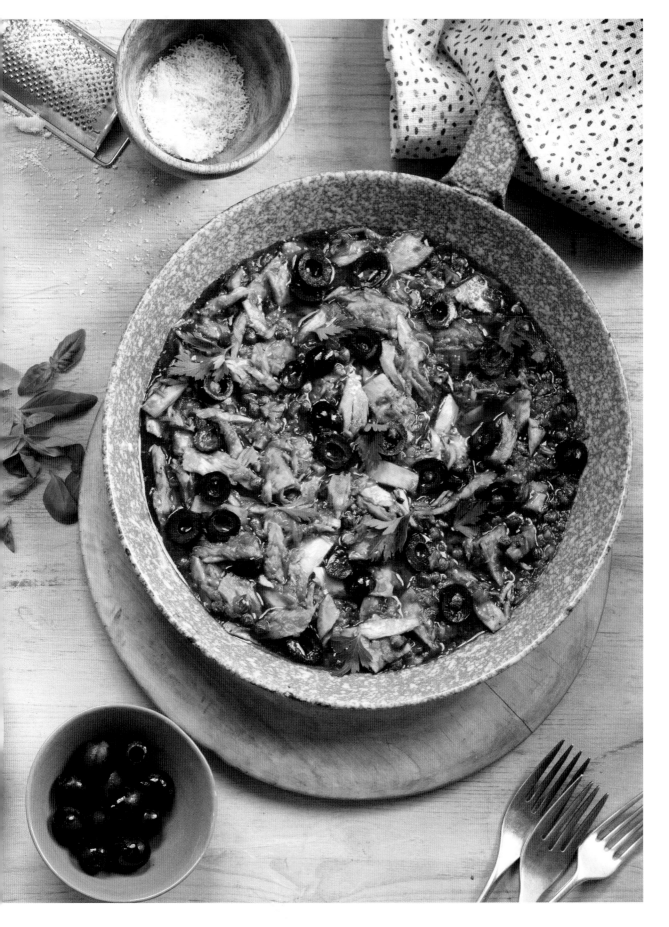

Blackened fish with bean and avocado salsa

Mmmm – this tropical salsa works beautifully with the spicy fish and the whole dish is ready in minutes. Add chips for the kids! My sweet potato fries (see page 160) always go down well.

1 First make the bean and avocado salsa. Mix all the ingredients in a bowl and season them with salt and black pepper. Leave the salsa to stand at room temperature while you cook the fish to allow the flavours time to blend.

2 Season the fish with salt on both sides. If using the spice mix, stir all the spices together in a bowl. Mix the flour with either the Cajun seasoning or the spice mix, then add a generous pinch of salt. Roll the fish fillets in the seasoned flour until they're thoroughly coated, then pat off any excess.

3 Heat the olive oil in a frying pan large enough to hold all the fish fillets. Add the fillets and fry them for 2–3 minutes on each side until they are well browned and just cooked through – thick fillets might need a little longer.

4 Serve the fish with the salsa on the side and wedges of limes to squeeze over the top if you fancy.

Serves 4

4 x 150g skinned fish fillets (such as tilapia or snapper)
50g wholemeal flour
2 tbsp Cajun seasoning or spice mix (see below)
1 tbsp olive oil
lime wedges, to serve
salt

Spice mix (optional)
1 tsp ground black pepper
1 tsp smoked paprika
1 tsp cayenne
1 tsp dried oregano
1 tsp garlic powder

Bean and avocado salsa
400g can of black beans, drained and rinsed
1 medium avocado, diced
1 medium mango, diced
3 spring onions, sliced into rounds
1 red chilli, deseeded and finely chopped
1 garlic clove, finely chopped
zest and juice of 1 lime
1 tbsp olive oil
salt and black pepper

427 calories per serving

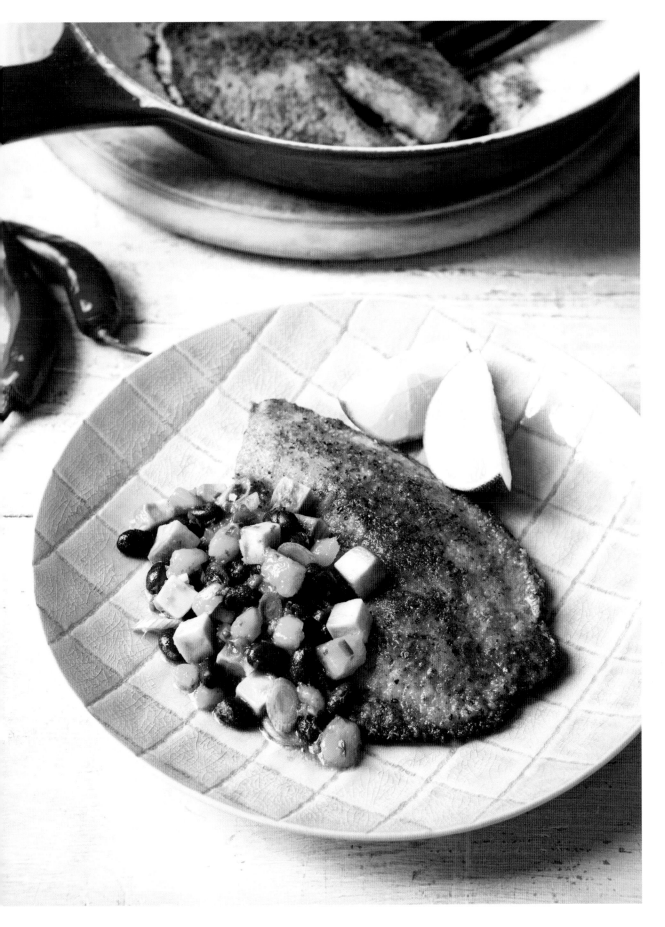

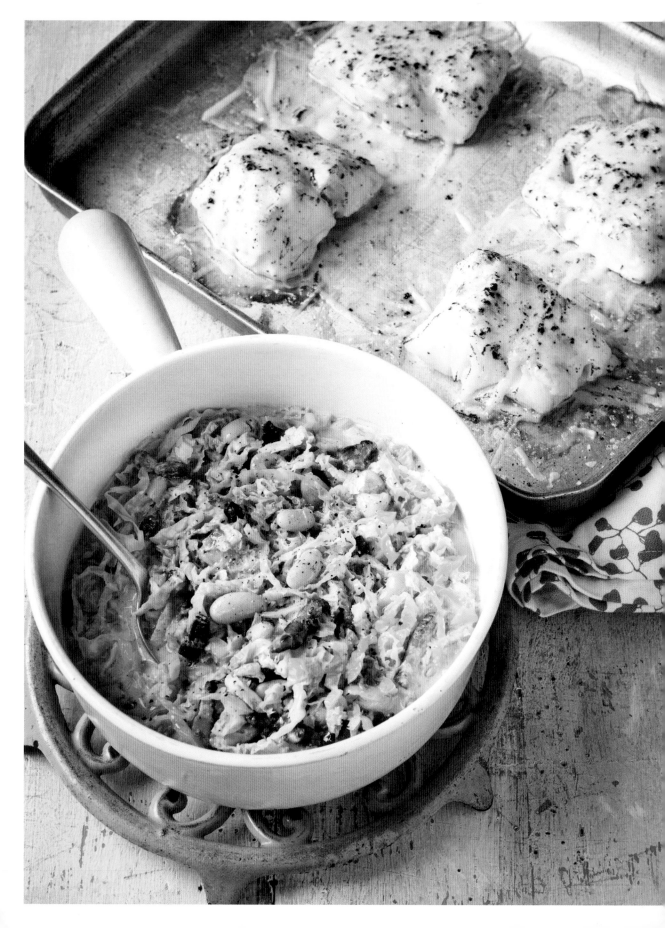

Roasted fish with braised cabbage and bacon

Not quite a one-pot, but this is a lovely complete meal that's ideal on a chilly autumn or winter evening. I like to use nice thick loin fillets – hake, cod or haddock all work well. A bit of mustard on the side is good if you're a fan.

1 Preheat the oven to 200°C/180°C Fan/Gas 6. Arrange the fish fillets on a baking tray, season them with salt and pepper and sprinkle the cheese on top. Put the tray in the oven and roast the fish for 20 minutes until it's just cooked through.

2 Meanwhile, heat the olive oil in a large, deep-sided frying pan that has a lid. Add the bacon and cook it over quite a high heat until crisp. Turn the heat down, add the onion and fry it gently until it has started to soften and turn golden brown.

3 Add the lemon zest, thyme and cabbage. Stir for a couple of minutes, pushing the cabbage well down into the pan, then pour the stock over the cabbage and sprinkle in the beans. Season with salt and pepper. Cover the pan and cook the cabbage for 5 minutes until it has collapsed down a little and is fairly soft, stirring occasionally. Stir in the crème fraiche and simmer, uncovered until the crème fraiche has combined with the stock.

4 Spoon the cabbage mixture into large, shallow bowls and serve with the fish on top.

Serves 4

4 x 150g white fish fillets (thick ones are best)
50g Cheddar or other hard cheese, grated
1 tsp olive oil
100g smoked bacon lardons
1 small onion, finely chopped
zest of 1 lemon
sprig of thyme, leaves only
1 small savoy cabbage, cored and shredded
200ml chicken or vegetable stock
400g can of cannellini beans, drained and rinsed
60ml crème fraiche
salt and black pepper

400 calories per serving

Chinese fish parcels

I really like this way of cooking fish. It's so easy and you can get the parcels all prepared, then pop them in the oven when you're ready. Let everyone open up their own little package of goodies at the table. With all the veggies, this does make a complete meal, but you can add some brown rice or noodles on the side for those who want more carbs. The carrot does up the carbs so we've left it optional, but I like to include it for colour and flavour.

1 Preheat the oven to 200°C/180°C Fan/Gas 6. Put a couple of baking trays in the oven to warm up – don't try to cram all the parcels on to one tray, as the fish will cook unevenly. Cut 4 large sheets of foil or baking parchment.

2 Season the fish with salt and black pepper. Divide the vegetables between each piece of foil or parchment, putting the baby corn on the bottom and building up to the carrot. Place a fillet of fish on top of each pile of vegetables, then sprinkle a tablespoon of soy sauce and a teaspoon of rice vinegar over each fillet. Sprinkle with the garlic, ginger, shallot and chillies.

3 Bring the sides of the parcel up and scrunch them together, then fold in the sides. Place the parcels on the heated baking trays and put them in the oven.

4 Cook for 12–15 minutes, depending on the thickness of the fish. If you've wrapped your parcels in parchment rather than foil the fish will cook slightly more quickly, so check the parcels after 12 minutes. You should find the fish is just cooked through and the vegetables will be perfectly done.

5 Serve the parcels with some sesame oil and a few coriander leaves for people to add if they like.

Serves 4

4 x 150g fish fillets (sea bream or other white fish)
150g–200g baby corn, sliced lengthways
100g mangetout
1 large courgette, cut into matchsticks
1 large carrot, cut into matchsticks (optional)
4 tbsp soy sauce
4 tsp rice vinegar
2 garlic cloves, finely sliced
10g fresh root ginger, finely chopped
1 shallot, thinly sliced
2 red chillies, thinly sliced
salt and black pepper

To serve
a few drops of sesame oil
coriander leaves

175 calories per serving

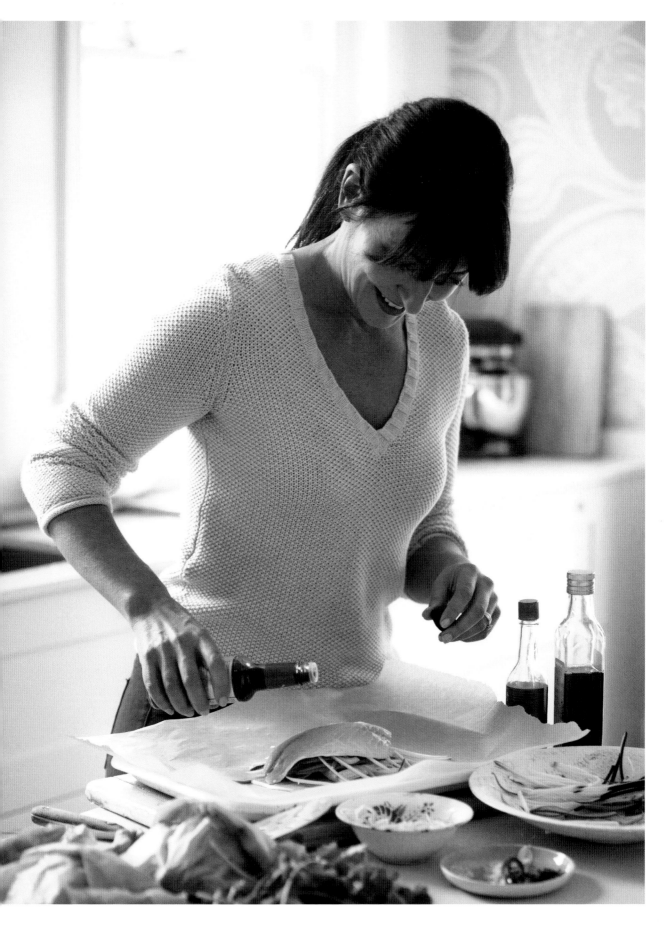

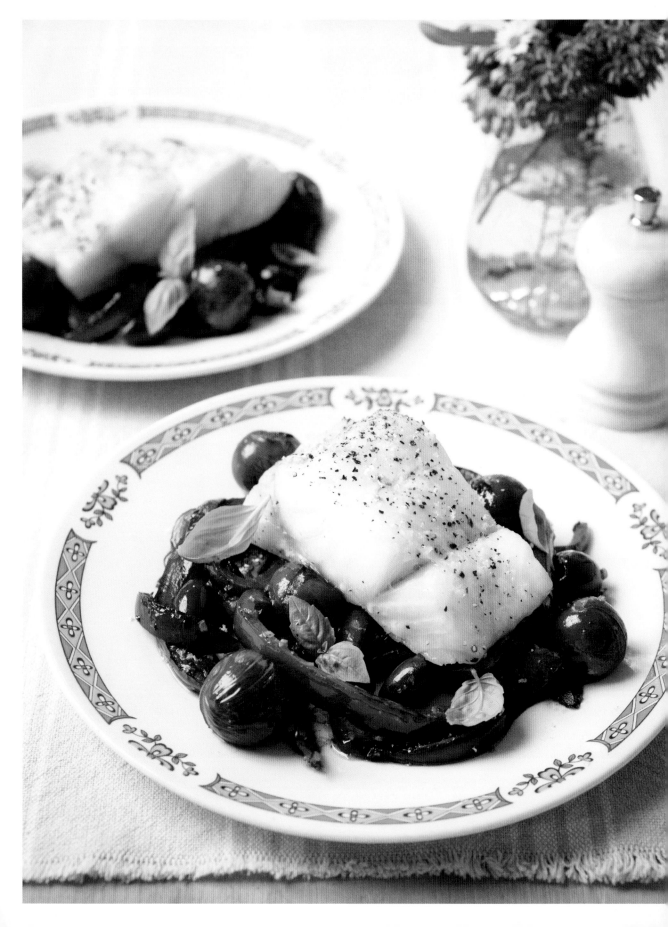

Fish Provençal

Simple, quick and tastes of sunshine – love it.

1 Preheat the oven to 200°C/180°C Fan/Gas 6. Season the fish fillets with salt and pepper and arrange them on a baking tray. Roast the fish in the oven for 10–12 minutes until it's cooked through.

2 Meanwhile, heat the oil in a large, shallow frying pan and add the red onion and red peppers. Cook them for 10 minutes over a medium heat until softened, stirring regularly. Add the garlic, lemon zest, olives and cherry tomatoes, then season with salt and pepper. Cover the pan and leave everything to cook gently over a low heat for 3–4 minutes, until the tomatoes have plumped up and are warmed through, but not burst.

3 Arrange the fish fillets and vegetables on 4 plates. Whisk the olive oil with the balsamic vinegar and drizzle this over the fish, then sprinkle over a few basil leaves.

Serves 4

4 x 150g chunky white fish fillets
  (cod or haddock both good)
1 tbsp olive oil
1 red onion, cut into thin wedges
2 red peppers, deseeded and sliced
  lengthways
2 garlic cloves, finely chopped
zest of 1 lemon
12 pitted black olives
200g cherry tomatoes, left whole
salt and black pepper

To serve
1 tbsp olive oil
1 tsp balsamic vinegar
a few basil leaves

217 calories per serving

Seafood tagine

This simple fish stew is all cooked in one pot and makes a great supper served with barley couscous, or my veggie couscous (see page 168) or just with a green salad. You could also add a little bit of preserved lemon – you can get it in supermarkets – towards the end of the cooking time for an authentic North African flavour. Any white fish is fine or you could buy the seafood mix you see on some fish counters. Don't get the one with smoked haddock, though, as the flavour isn't right for this dish.

1 Heat the olive oil in a large casserole dish, then add the onion and fennel. Add a splash of water, put a lid on the dish and cook over a low heat for about 10 minutes, stirring regularly, until the onion and fennel are starting to look translucent.

2 Add the garlic, spices and lemon zest and stir for a minute or so to coat the vegetables. Pour the saffron strands with their water and the stock into the dish, then season with salt and pepper. Bring the liquid to the boil, turn down the heat to a low simmer and cover the dish again. Cook for about 10 minutes until the fennel is completely tender.

3 Add the fish and prawns to the tagine and cook for a couple of minutes until the prawns are pink and the fish has turned an opaque white. Add half the lemon juice, then taste and add the rest if you think the dish needs it.

4 Sprinkle with the herbs before serving.

Serves 4

1 tbsp olive oil
1 small onion, finely chopped
2 small bulbs of fennel, sliced
    lengthways into thin wedges
2 garlic cloves, finely chopped
½ tsp turmeric
½ tsp ground ginger
¼ tsp ground cinnamon
¼ tsp cayenne or chilli powder
zest and juice of 1 lemon
generous pinch of saffron strands,
    soaked in 2 tbsp hot water
600ml fish or vegetable stock
600g firm white fish, skinned, filleted
    and cut into chunks
12 raw tiger prawns, shelled and
    deveined
2 tbsp each of chopped coriander,
    parsley and mint leaves
salt and black pepper

198 calories per serving

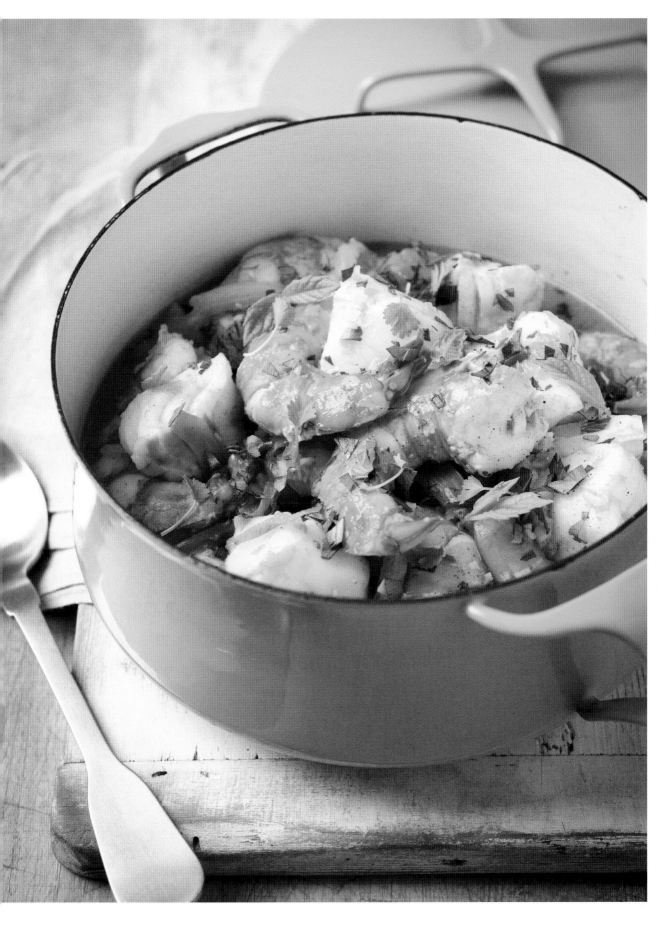

My Faves

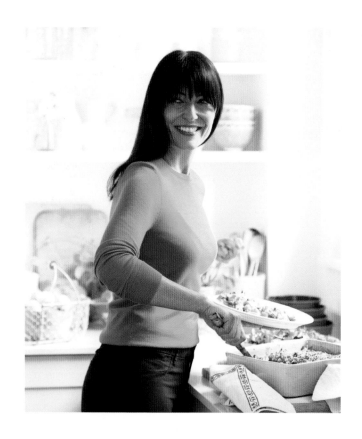

Chapter 5

Poultry + Meat

"More family favourites – so good you'll forget you're dieting and you won't feel hungry!"

Spanish chicken

Dishes like this make me think of wonderful sunny Mediterranean holidays. Cook up some veggie couscous (see page 168) to serve alongside if you like and there's supper sorted. You could pop in a bit of chorizo if you like but don't forget it will add extra calories.

1 Heat the olive oil in a large frying pan that has a lid. Fry the chicken over a high heat until it's browned on all sides. Remove the chicken with a slotted spoon and set it aside.

2 Add the onions and peppers and fry them briskly for a couple of minutes over a high heat, then turn down the heat, add about 50ml of water and cover the pan. Leave the veg to cook for 10 minutes until they've softened but are still keeping their shape.

3 Add the garlic and cook it for a couple of minutes, then put the chicken back in the pan. Add the saffron to the chicken stock, then pour this over the vegetables and chicken and season with the paprika and some salt and black pepper.

4 Bring the liquid to the boil, then turn down the heat to a gentle simmer and add the olives, capers, lemon zest and juice. Cook, uncovered, for about 10 minutes until the chicken is cooked through and the sauce is well reduced. Serve garnished with lots of parsley and basil leaves.

Serves 4

1 tbsp olive oil
600g skinless chicken thigh fillets, trimmed of fat and cut into strips
2 red onions, cut into wedges
2 large red peppers, cut into strips
2 garlic cloves, finely chopped
½ tsp saffron, soaked in 2 tbsp boiling water
300ml chicken stock
½ tsp sweet smoked paprika
50g pitted green olives, halved
25g capers, rinsed
zest and juice of 1 lemon
salt and black pepper

To serve
chopped parsley leaves
basil leaves

220 calories per serving

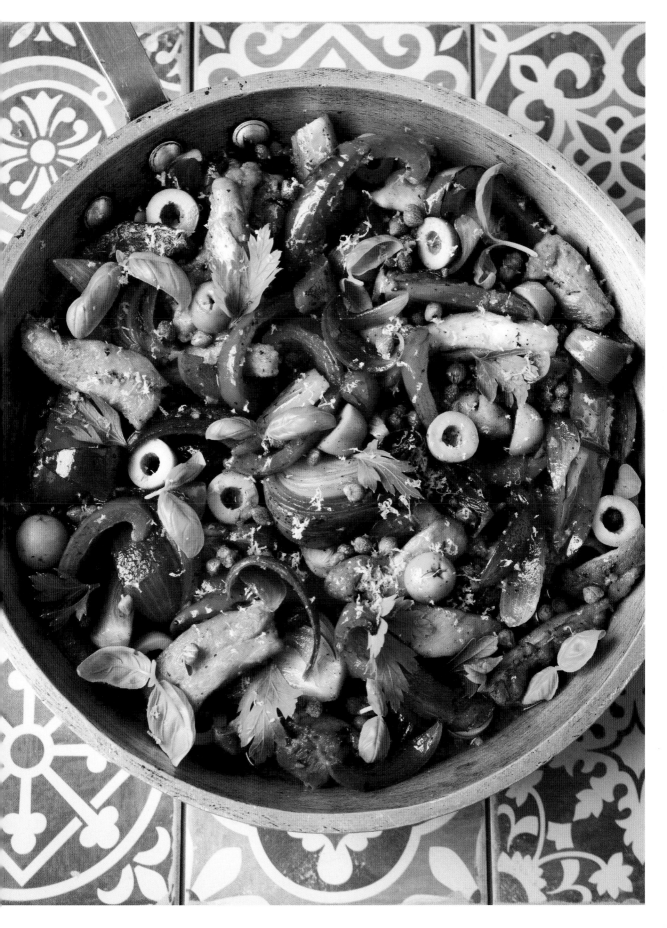

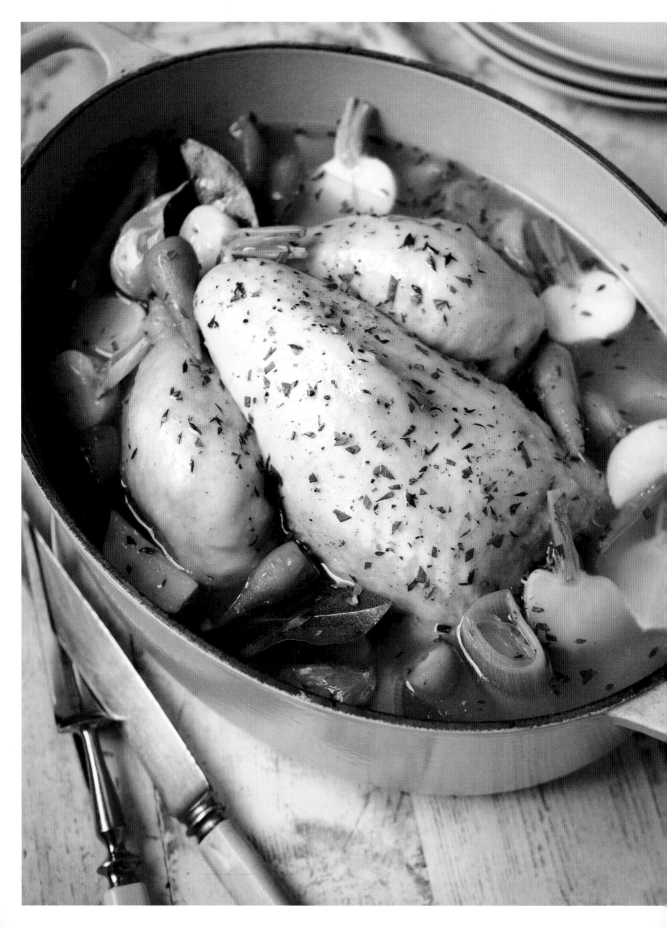

Poached chicken with lemon sauce

This is one of my sister Caroline's recipes. The children weren't keen at first because the chicken didn't look all golden and roasted, but once they'd tasted it they all went very quiet!!! Now it's another family fave.

1 Put the chicken in a large saucepan or a casserole dish – it should be a fairly snug fit. Break up the garlic and drop the unpeeled cloves into the pot, together with the lemon peel and herbs. Pour the stock or water into the pan and season with salt and pepper.

2 Bring the liquid to the boil, then turn the heat down to a fairly gentle simmer and cover the pan. Leave the chicken to cook for half an hour, then add the vegetables. Simmer for another 15 minutes, then remove the pan from the heat. Leave the chicken to stand for 15 minutes – it will continue to cook during this time.

3 Check the chicken is done – the juices in the thickest part of the leg should run clear. (If necessary, you can put the pan back over the heat for another 5 minutes or so.) Leave the chicken in the casserole dish, and ladle 400ml of the cooking liquid into a small saucepan.

4 Add the lemon peel to the reserved cooking liquid and boil until the liquid is reduced by half. Add the lemon juice and simmer for a couple of minutes to combine. Taste for seasoning and add salt and pepper if necessary. Whisk in the crème fraiche and simmer the sauce for another couple of minutes – it should be the consistency of single cream. Stir in the tarragon, if using.

5 Transfer the chicken to a platter, draining off any liquid that's collected inside. Arrange the vegetables and garlic cloves around the chicken and serve moistened with a small amount of the cooking liquid and the lemon sauce.

Serves 4

1 x 1.5–1.8kg chicken
1 bulb of garlic
2 thinly pared strips of lemon peel
3 bay leaves
1 large sprig of tarragon (optional)
1 large sprig of thyme
1.5 litres chicken stock or water
250g small carrots, peeled but
    left whole
2 turnips, cut into wedges
3 leeks, cut into rounds of 4–5cm
salt and black pepper

Sauce

1 thinly pared strip of lemon peel
juice of ½ lemon
50ml crème fraiche
leaves from a sprig of tarragon,
    finely chopped (optional)

386 calories per serving

Chicken crumble

This is totally amazing and such a perfect family supper. The topping is really crunchy and comforting but still low in calories so you can afford to help yourself to a generous portion. Love it.

1 Cut the chicken into chunks and dust them with the flour. Heat the olive oil in a large saucepan and fry the chicken until it's all well browned. It's best to do this in a couple of batches so you don't overcrowd the pan. Set each batch aside when it's ready.

2 Melt the butter in the pan, then add the squash and leeks. Stir until the vegetables are coated with butter, then sprinkle in the sage and season with salt and pepper. Pour in 300ml of stock, reserving the rest for cooking the quinoa.

3 Bring the stock to the boil, then turn down the heat and leave it to simmer for 7 minutes. Add the browned chicken and cook for another 5 minutes. By this point the vegetables should be almost tender and the chicken will be cooked through.

4 Using a slotted spoon, transfer the chicken and vegetables to an ovenproof dish. Bring the cooking liquid back to the boil and continue to cook until it's reduced by half. Add the crème fraiche and simmer for a few minutes until you have a sauce with the consistency of single cream. Pour this over the chicken and vegetables in the dish. Preheat the oven to 200°C/180°C Fan/Gas 6.

5 For the topping, put the quinoa in a saucepan and toast it over a medium heat. Pour over the reserved chicken stock and season it with salt. Bring the stock to the boil, then turn the heat down, cover the pan and leave the quinoa to simmer for 15 minutes. Remove the pan from the heat and leave the quinoa to stand for 5 minutes.

6 Divide the cauliflower into florets and blitz them in a food processor until they resemble breadcrumbs. Heat half the butter in a large frying pan. Add the cauliflower and the cooked quinoa and fry them for at least 5 minutes, until everything starts to turn a light golden brown. Stir in the Parmesan and parsley, then check the seasoning.

7 Sprinkle the topping over the chicken filling, then dot over the rest of the butter. Put the dish in the oven and bake for 30 minutes until the topping has browned round the edges and the filling is piping hot.

Serves 4

600g boneless, skinless chicken thigh or breast fillets, trimmed of fat
1 tbsp wholemeal spelt flour
1 tbsp olive oil
15g butter
500g butternut squash, diced
3 leeks, sliced
1 tsp dried sage
550ml chicken stock
1 tbsp crème fraiche
salt and black pepper

Topping
100g quinoa, well rinsed
250g cauliflower
10g butter
15g Parmesan cheese, grated
2 tbsp finely chopped parsley

471 calories per serving

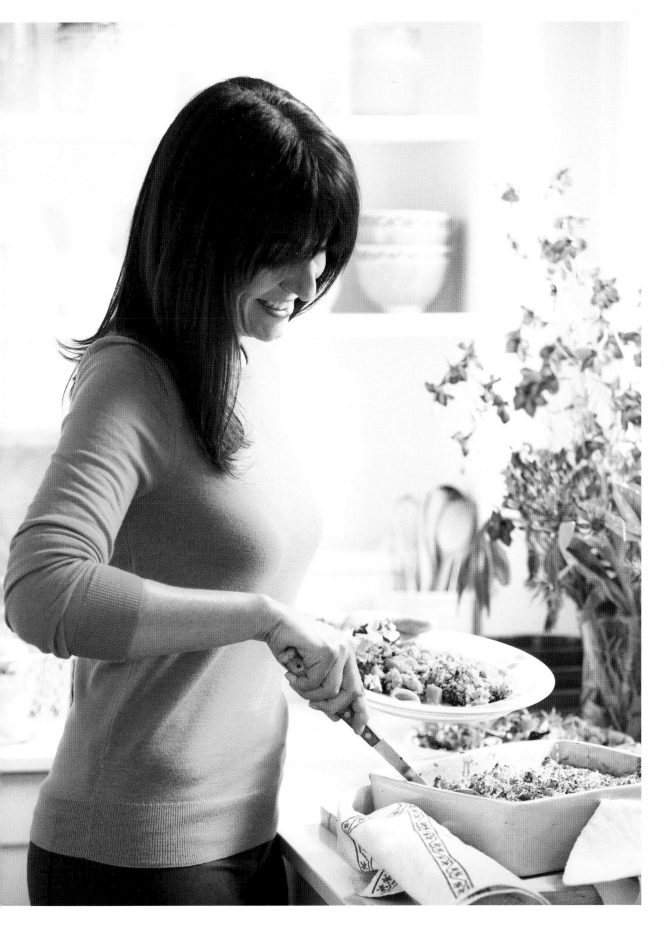

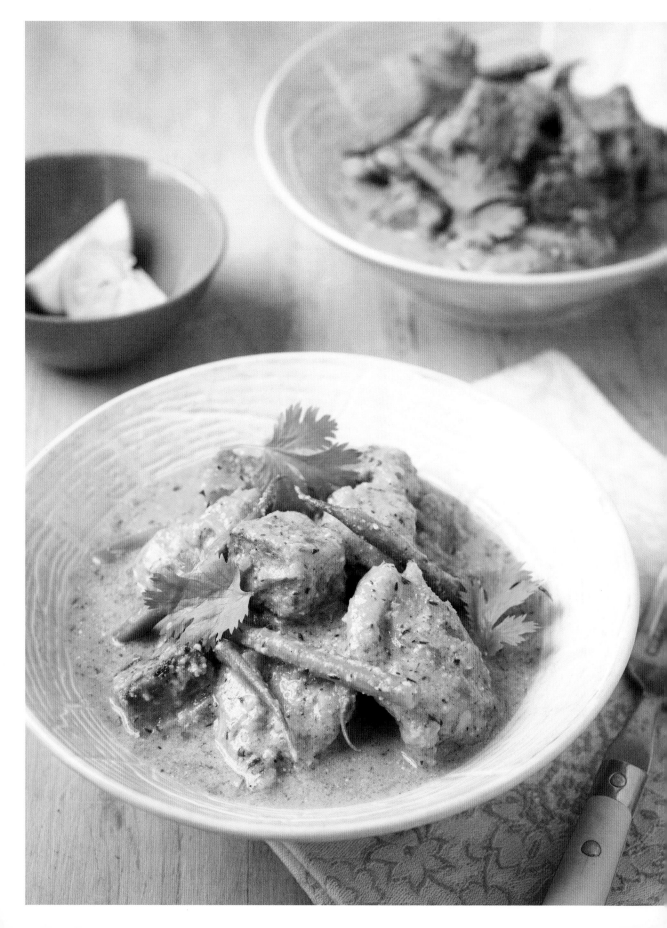

Chicken curry

I'd never thought of putting ground almonds into a curry but they work brilliantly and give it a nice mild sweet flavour. A good yellow curry powder is fine here or if you have *5 Weeks to Sugar-Free*, use my spice mix recipe.

1 Heat the oil in a large casserole dish or a saucepan. Add the sliced onion and cook it over a low heat until it's soft and translucent, then add the garlic and cook for another minute or so.

2 Add the curry powder or spice mix and ground almonds and stir for another couple of minutes, then add the chicken. Stir to coat the chicken with the spice and almonds, then add the chicken stock, bay leaves and butternut squash. Season with salt and pepper.

3 Cover the dish or pan and simmer for about 10 minutes, then add the green beans. Continue to cook for 5 minutes, still covered, then remove the lid and stir in the yoghurt. Simmer for another 5 minutes until the sauce has thickened slightly, making sure it doesn't boil.

4 Serve with lime wedges and a sprinkling of coriander leaves.

Serves 4

1 tbsp vegetable or coconut oil
1 onion, finely sliced
2 garlic cloves, finely chopped
2 tbsp mild yellow curry powder
    or spice mix
50g ground almonds
600g boneless, skinless chicken
    thighs or breasts, trimmed of
    fat and diced
300ml chicken stock
2 bay leaves
200g butternut squash, cut into
    large dice
100g green beans, topped
50ml Greek yoghurt
salt and black pepper

To serve
lime wedges
a few coriander leaves

337 calories per serving

Grilled chicken with tahini sauce

Butterflying chicken breasts just means cutting them in half through the middle so they are thinner and cook quickly. Easy peasy. If the chicken breasts are large you may find that two is enough to feed four, particularly if you're serving something on the side. Love the tahini sauce – tahini is a paste made from sesame seeds and you can buy it, and pomegranate molasses, in supermarkets.

1 First butterfly the chicken breasts. Put one on a flat surface, then, keeping it steady with one hand, hold your knife parallel to the work surface and cut through the breast from one side to the other, stopping short of cutting right the way through. You will then be able to open out the breast like a book and press it flat along the join. Repeat with the other breasts and put them all in a shallow dish.

2 Season the chicken breasts with salt and pepper, then dilute the lemon juice with the same amount of water and pour it over the chicken breasts. Leave them to stand for a few minutes.

3 Preheat a griddle pan until it's very hot, then grill the chicken breasts for 3–4 minutes on each side until cooked through and marked with brown char lines. Leave them to rest for a few minutes.

4 To make the sauce, put all the ingredients in a blender and season with salt and pepper. Add 100ml of water and blitz until the sauce is fairly smooth and flecked with green.

5 Serve the chicken with a drizzle of the sauce and a sprinkling of herbs and pomegranate seeds. A salad on the side is nice and perhaps some braised barley (see page 163).

Serves 4

4 skinless, boneless chicken breasts
juice of 1 lemon
salt and black pepper

Tahini sauce
100g tahini, well stirred
juice of 2 lemons
1 tbsp pomegranate molasses
    (optional)
2 garlic cloves, crushed
1 tsp ground cumin
small bunch of parsley, finely
    chopped
small bunch of coriander, finely
    chopped

To serve
parsley and coriander leaves
pomegranate seeds (optional)

320 calories per serving

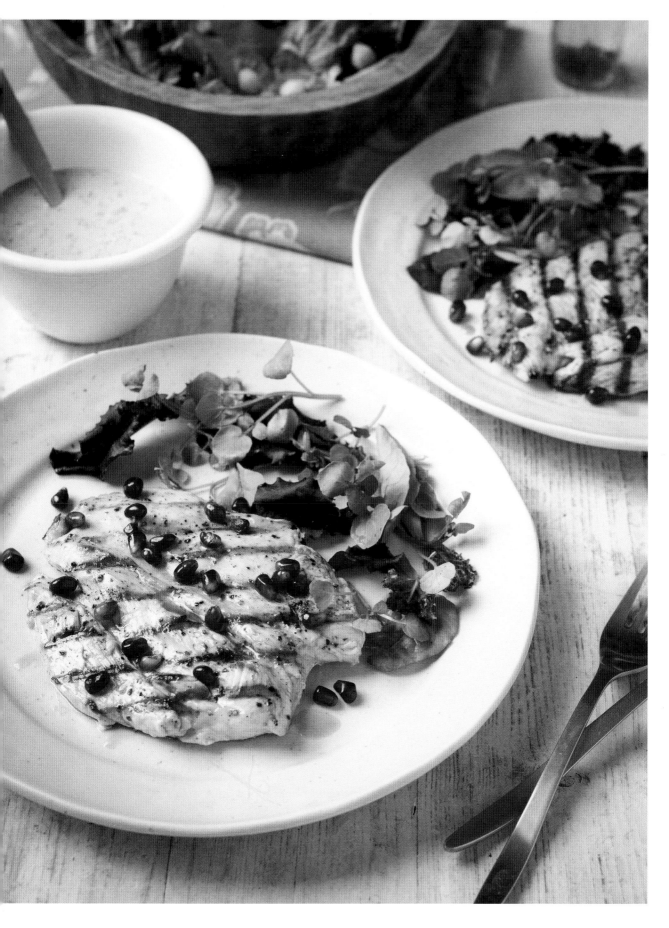

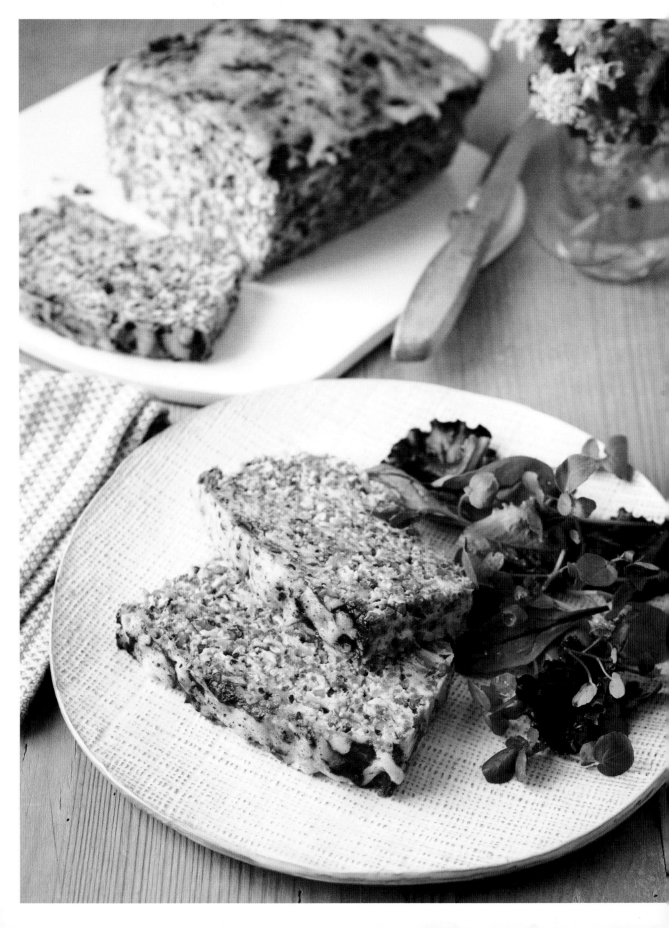

Chicken meatloaf

Many meatloaf recipes contain sugary tomato ketchup which I prefer to avoid – unless it's the sugar-free sort I have a recipe for in *5 Weeks to Sugar-Free*. This version is made with tomato purée instead, but I put a special maple syrup glaze over it that the children love. You can also make this meatloaf with turkey mince.

1 Preheat the oven to 180°C/160°C Fan/Gas 4. Line a 1kg loaf tin with foil and spray the foil lightly with olive oil.

2 Put the chicken mince in a large bowl. Add the onion, mushrooms, garlic, cooked quinoa and herbs, and season with salt and pepper.

3 Mix 2 tablespoons of the tomato purée with the chicken stock, then add this and the egg to the chicken mixture. Mix thoroughly – it's best to do this with your hands. Pile the mixture into the prepared tin and smooth it down, then bake the meatloaf in the oven for 30 minutes.

4 Mix the remaining tomato purée with the Worcestershire sauce, maple syrup and grated cheese. Take the meatloaf out of the oven, spread it with the maple syrup mixture, then pop it back into the oven for 10 minutes.

5 Serve in slices with some vegetables or salad. Some home-made tomato sauce goes really well with this too.

Serves 4–6

olive oil spray
750g chicken mince
1 small onion, finely chopped
100g white or chestnut mushrooms, finely chopped
1 garlic clove, finely chopped
200g cooked quinoa (see p.204)
1 tsp dried oregano
2 tbsp finely chopped parsley
4 tbsp tomato purée
50ml chicken stock
1 egg, beaten
dash of Worcestershire sauce
1 tsp maple syrup
50g Cheddar cheese, grated
salt and black pepper

*393 calories per portion
if serving 4; 262 if serving 6*

Vietnamese chicken stir-fry

Get everything chopped and sliced and trimmed, then this is so quick to make – and tastes amazing. You could add some noodles for anyone who's not calorie and carb counting. Fish sauce and lemongrass might sound a bit exotic but you'll find them in all the supermarkets now.

1 Put the slices of chicken in a bowl and season them with salt and pepper. Add the lime zest and half the lime juice, then stir briefly to combine. Peel the outer layers off the lemongrass stalks and slice the white inner core into thin rounds.

2 Heat the oil in a wok. When the oil is very hot (you can tell, as it starts to shimmer slightly) add the lemongrass, garlic and ginger. Stir for 30 seconds, then drain the chicken and add this too. Stir-fry the chicken slices for a moment to brown them, then sprinkle in the turmeric and add the mushrooms, green beans and sprouting broccoli.

3 Continue to stir-fry until the vegetables are just cooked and the beans and broccoli are still fairly crisp. Check for seasoning and add the remaining lime juice and the fish sauce.

4 Sprinkle with the spring onions, chillies and herbs before serving.

Serves 4

600g skinless, boneless chicken breasts or thighs, trimmed of fat and thinly sliced
zest of 1 lime
juice of 2 limes
2 lemongrass stalks
1 tbsp vegetable or coconut oil
2 garlic cloves, finely chopped
10g fresh root ginger, finely chopped
½ tsp ground turmeric
200g button mushrooms, halved
100g green beans, topped and halved
200g sprouting broccoli, trimmed and cut in half
1 tbsp fish sauce (nam pla)
salt and black pepper

To serve
2 spring onions, halved and shredded lengthways
2 red or green chillies, deseeded and sliced into rounds
handful of coriander leaves
handful of Thai (or regular) basil leaves
handful of mint leaves

223 calories per serving

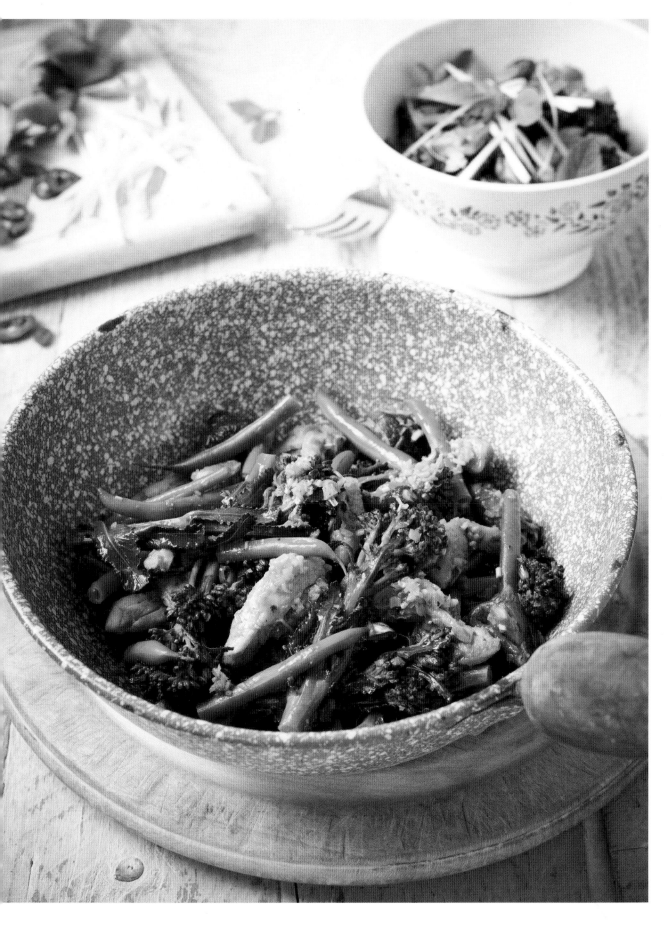

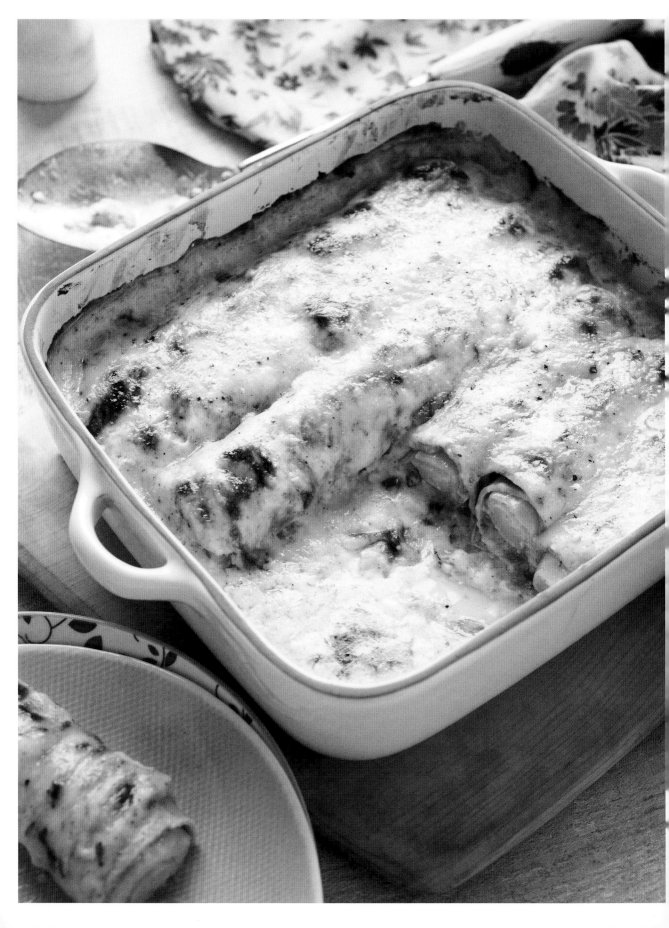

Leek and ham gratin

I know, this looks soooo naughty! But it's not *too* naughty because we've kept the quantity of cheese down and spiced things up with a bit of mustard. Great meal for the fam.

1 Make sure all the leeks are well trimmed and thoroughly cleaned. Melt the butter in a pan wide enough to hold the leeks in a single layer. Add the leeks and turn them until they're coated in the butter, then add 200ml of water. Bring the water to the boil, then turn the heat down to a very low simmer and cover the pan.

2 Leave the leeks to cook gently for 8–10 minutes, turning them every so often, until they are just tender when pierced with a knife, but in no danger of collapsing. Remove the pan from the heat and allow the leeks to cool.

3 Spread the mustard over the slices of ham, then wrap each piece of leek in a slice of ham. Lightly butter an ovenproof dish and arrange the wrapped leeks in it. Preheat the oven to 200°C/180°C Fan/Gas 6.

4 Now make the béchamel sauce. Melt the butter in a small pan, add the flour and stir for a couple of minutes to cook out the raw flavour.

5 Add the milk, about 100ml at a time, stirring constantly between additions to avoid lumps. When all the milk is incorporated, you should have a fairly runny sauce. Turn the heat up slightly and keep stirring until the sauce gets close to boiling point and starts to thicken. Season with salt and pepper.

6 Pour the béchamel sauce over the leeks, then top with the grated cheese. Put the dish in the oven and bake for 20–25 minutes until the cheese has browned and the sauce is bubbling.

Serves 4

6 large leeks, cut in half
10g butter, plus extra for greasing
1 tbsp Dijon or English mustard
12 thin slices of ham
25g Gruyère or similar hard cheese, grated

Béchamel sauce

25g butter
25g wholemeal or wholemeal spelt flour
400ml whole milk
salt and black pepper

303 calories per serving

Slow-roast pork with braised fennel

Pork roasted really, really slowly is the most delicious thing ever. It can be fatty though, but in this method you pour off most of the fat before the end of the cooking time, so reducing the calorie count while keeping lots of flavour. This does take some time to cook so start early!

1 Preheat the oven to 150°C/130°C Fan/Gas 2. Place the pork in a large roasting tin, rub it with a little oil, then sprinkle it with salt. Pour in 300ml of just-boiled water, then cover the whole roasting tin with foil.

2 Put the pork in the oven and roast it for 4 hours. Remove the tin from the oven, carefully remove the foil and set the meat aside on a board for a few moments. Strain off all the fat and liquid from the tin into a bowl and set it aside to cool.

3 Put the sliced onions and fennel wedges in the roasting tin, trying to make sure most of the fennel is in the centre, then season them with salt and pepper. Put the pork back on top of the vegetables and add another 200ml of just-boiled water. Cover the tin with foil again and roast for a further 2 hours.

4 Turn the oven temperature up to 220°C/200°C Fan/Gas 7. Remove the foil and add 300ml of just-boiled water to the tin. Continue to roast the pork at the higher heat for another 45 minutes to crisp up the skin.

5 Take the pork out of the oven and put it on a serving platter or board. Cover it loosely with foil and leave it to rest for 20 minutes. Remove the vegetables and keep them warm.

6 Remove any fat from the cooled, reserved cooking liquid. Add the cooking liquid to any juices in the roasting tin and heat it through, then pour it all into a warm gravy boat. Take the skin (crackling) off the pork before carving if you like and serve it separately.

Serves 4

1 boned and rolled pork shoulder, skin scored (about 2.5kg)
1 tbsp olive oil
2 red onions, sliced
2 fennel bulbs, trimmed and cut into thin wedges
salt and black pepper

480 calories per serving; 411 without crackling

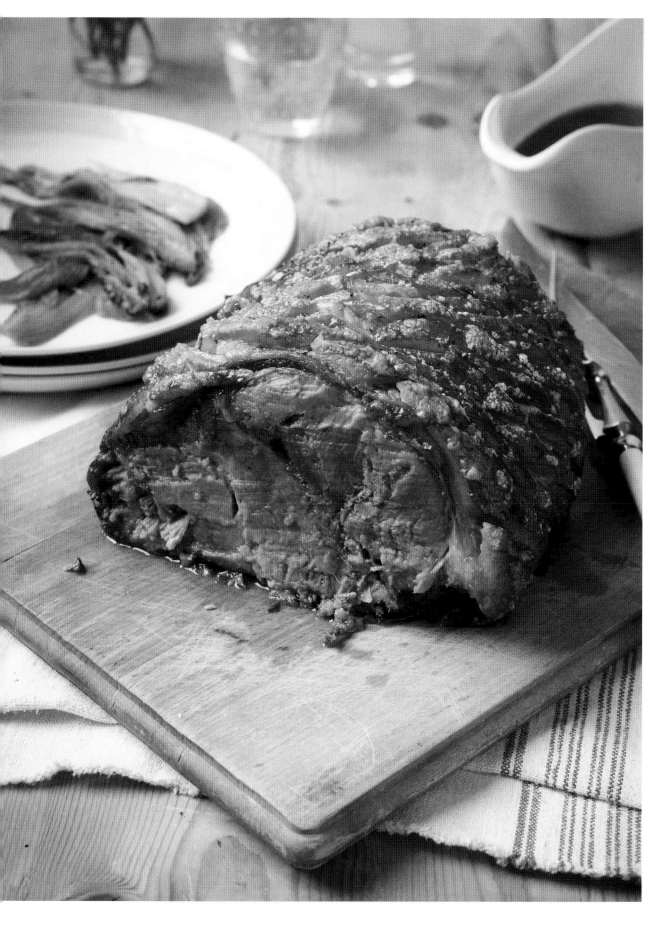

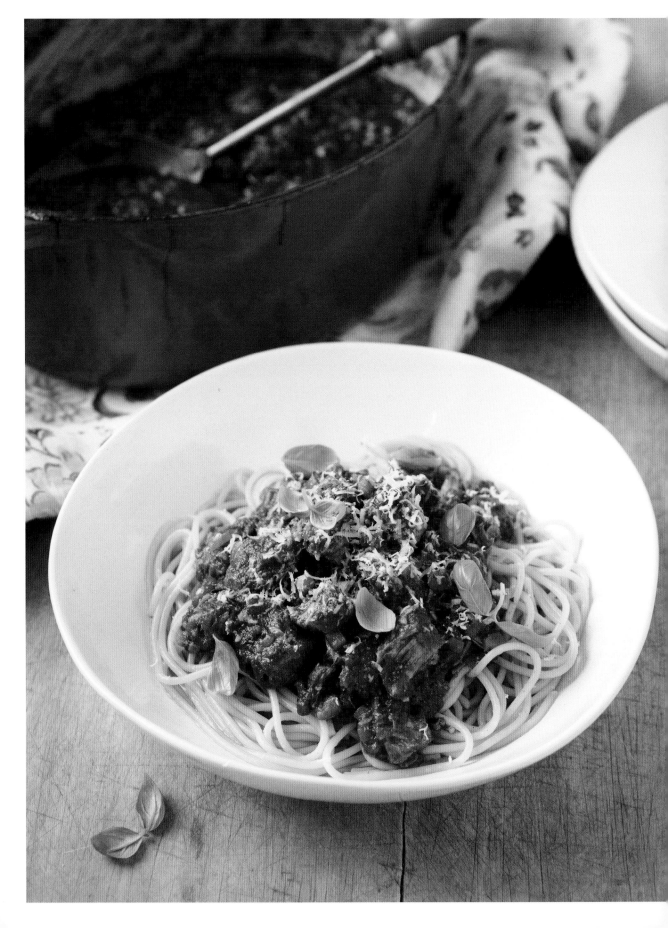

Pork ragu

This is based on an amazing pasta dish I ate in France and completely loved. The sauce is cooked for ages over a low heat until the meat is falling apart – so good. It's worth making lots and stashing it away in the freezer if you don't use it all. If you don't have the fresh herbs you could use dried herbes de Provence instead or some Italian dried herbs.

1 Heat a tablespoon of the oil in a large frying pan and fry the diced pork shoulder until it's well browned on all sides. It's best to do this in batches so you don't overcrowd the pan or the meat will stew, not brown. Set each batch aside as it's browned.

2 Meanwhile, heat the remaining olive oil in a large casserole dish. Add the onion, celery and carrots and fry them gently for several minutes over a fairly low heat until they've started to soften. Add the garlic and herbs, then cook for another couple of minutes.

3 Add the browned pork to the casserole dish, then add a little of the wine, if using, or some water to the frying pan and scrape up any brown bits. Tip this into the casserole, then add the rest of the wine, if using, and turn up the heat. Boil fiercely until the wine has evaporated, then add the tomatoes and season with salt and pepper.

4 Bring the mixture back to the boil, then turn down the heat and cover the casserole dish with a lid. Simmer very gently for at least an hour and a half, or until the pork is starting to shred and is very tender.

5 Take the lid off the casserole dish and leave it over a low heat until the sauce has reduced down. Stir occasionally to help shred the meat and help it combine with the rest of the sauce.

6 Remove the sprigs of herbs, then serve the sauce with pasta or some grated Parmesan. You can also serve the sauce with spiralised courgettes for a lower calorie count.

Serves 6–8

2 tbsp olive oil
1kg boned pork shoulder, trimmed
    of fat and cut into 3–4cm dice
1 large onion, finely diced
2 celery sticks, finely chopped
2 carrots, finely chopped
3 garlic cloves, finely chopped
1 large sprig of rosemary, left whole
1 large sprig of thyme, left whole
1 large sprig of sage, left whole
2 bay leaves
250ml white wine (optional)
2 x 400g cans of chopped tomatoes
salt and black pepper

To serve
50g wholewheat pasta
grated Parmesan cheese (optional)

472 calories per portion
if serving 6; 400 if serving 8

Lamb and aubergine casserole

Good with some veggie couscous (see page 168) on the side. If you like, you can use a spice mix, such as ras el hanout, instead of the spices listed.

1 Preheat the oven to 220°C/200°C Fan/Gas 7. Put the aubergines in a bowl and spritz them with olive oil spray, then turn them over and repeat. Spread the aubergines on a baking tray and roast them in the oven for about 20 minutes, until they're starting to brown.

2 Heat the olive oil in a large flameproof casserole dish. Add the sliced onion and cook it slowly over a gentle heat for about 10 minutes, until it's soft and translucent, then turn up the heat and add the lamb. Cook until the lamb is well browned, stirring regularly, then reduce the heat and add the garlic and spices. Season with salt and pepper.

3 Add the tomatoes and the stock or water. Bring to the boil, then turn down the heat, put a lid on the casserole dish and simmer for an hour until the lamb is becoming tender. Add the aubergines and the pomegranate molasses, cover again and cook for another 30 minutes.

4 Remove the lid from the casserole. If the sauce is very liquid, simmer until it has reduced slightly, then add the lemon juice. Serve sprinkled with parsley.

Serves 4

2 aubergines, cut into 2.5cm cubes
olive oil spray
1 tbsp olive oil
1 large onion, finely sliced
600g lean lamb leg or shoulder, trimmed of fat and diced
2 garlic cloves, finely chopped
½ tsp ground allspice
½ tsp ground cumin
½ tsp ground coriander
½ tsp cayenne or hot chilli powder
¼ tsp ground cinnamon
400g can of chopped tomatoes
200ml chicken stock or water
1 tbsp pomegranate molasses
1 tbsp lemon juice
small bunch of parsley, leaves only, to serve
salt and black pepper

334 calories per serving

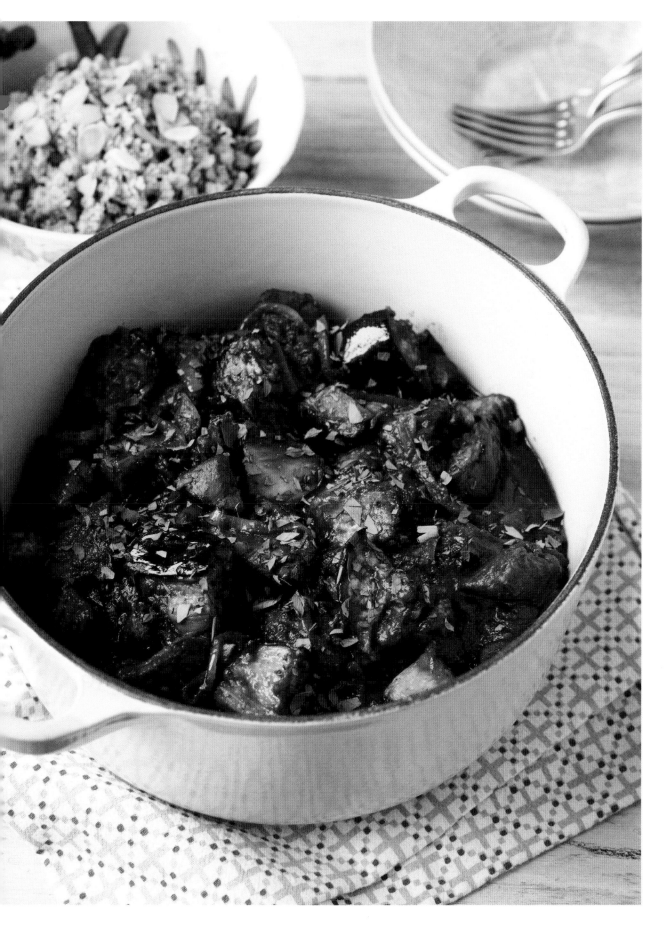

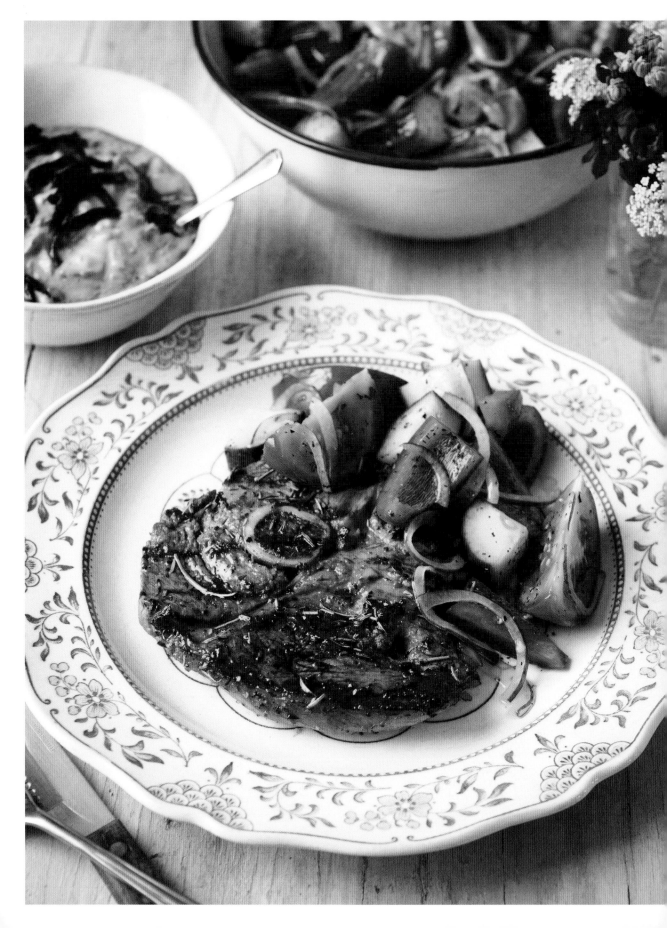

Greek lamb

Eating this combo is like being on holiday – it's so full of sunny flavour and colour. Ask for fairly thin lamb steaks so they're not too high in calories and they cook quickly. The beetroot tzatziki is sensational, but if you're not a beetroot fan, just use cucumber.

1 Put the lamb steaks in a bag or bowl. Add the olive oil, lemon juice and zest, garlic and herbs, then season with salt and pepper. Leave the meat to marinate for as long as you can but for at least an hour.

2 To make the tzatziki, put the yoghurt in a bowl and add the beetroot. Peel, deseed and grate the cucumber, then strain it in a sieve, squeezing out any excess water. Add the cucumber to the yoghurt along with the garlic and mint, then season with salt and pepper. Set the tzatziki aside until you're ready to eat.

3 To make the salad, put the tomatoes, cucumber, pepper and onion in a bowl. Season with salt and pepper and sprinkle with the herbs, then drizzle over the olive oil and red wine vinegar.

4 When you are ready to cook the lamb, heat a griddle pan until it's very hot. Cook the lamb steaks for a couple of minutes on each side or until black char lines appear. Leave the meat to rest for 5 minutes before serving with the tzatziki and Greek salad.

Serves 4

4 x 150g lamb steaks, trimmed of fat
1 tbsp olive oil
juice and zest of 1 lemon
2 garlic cloves, thinly sliced
1 tbsp mixed Mediterranean herbs
    (oregano, thyme, rosemary, sage)
salt and black pepper

Beetroot tzatziki
200g Greek yoghurt
1 cooked beetroot (about 75g), grated
½ cucumber
1 garlic clove, finely chopped
½ tsp dried mint

Greek salad
4 tomatoes, quartered
½ cucumber, cut into chunks
1 red or green pepper, cut into slices
1 small red onion, sliced
½ tsp dried oregano or mixed herbs
1 tbsp olive oil
1 tsp red wine vinegar

387 calories per serving

Beef casserole with squash and chestnut dumplings

There's nothing like a beef casserole on a winter evening. Yes, it does need to be cooked for a while but it's not difficult to make and once it's in the oven you can relax, knowing supper is on the way. The dumplings are made with chestnuts and butternut squash instead of suet and stodge and they are crazy tasty; a real crowd pleaser.

1 Heat a tablespoon of the olive oil in a large flameproof casserole dish or a saucepan. Add the onion, celery and carrots and cook them for several minutes over a medium heat until they're starting to brown. At the same time, heat the remaining olive oil in a large frying pan and sear the steak on all sides until it's all well browned. It's best to do this in a couple of batches so you don't overcrowd the pan, setting each batch aside as it is browned.

2 Add the garlic to the casserole dish and cook it gently for a couple of minutes, then add the beef. If using the wine, use some of it to deglaze the frying pan, scraping up any brown bits and pouring them over the beef. If not using wine, use a little water instead.

3 Add the remaining wine and the stock to the casserole dish, tuck in the herbs and season with salt and pepper. Bring to the boil, then turn down the heat, cover and leave to simmer gently for a couple of hours, until the beef is tender.

4 To make the dumplings, sift the flour into a bowl with the baking powder, sage and a generous amount of salt and pepper. Grate half the chestnuts and add these too, then crumble in the rest. Squeeze out as much of the liquid from the butternut squash as you can, then add it to the bowl together with the butter. Mix thoroughly until everything is completely combined. You will have a fairly soft mixture which will be quite easy to roll into 8 balls.

5 Take the lid off the dish and drop the dumplings on top. Put the lid back on and leave everything to simmer for another 15-20 minutes. The dumplings will be well risen, light and fluffy. Remove the casserole from the heat and serve immediately with some green veg on the side.

Serves 4–6

2 tbsp olive oil
1 large onion, cut into thin
    wedges
2 celery sticks, sliced
2 carrots, cut into diagonal slices
800g stewing steak, trimmed and
    cut into 4cm pieces
2 garlic cloves, finely chopped
250ml red wine (optional)
up to 500ml beef stock
    (250ml if using the wine)
sprig of thyme
1 tsp dried sage
2 bay leaves
salt and black pepper

Dumplings
100g wholemeal spelt flour
1 tsp baking powder
½ tsp sage
150g vacuum-packed chestnuts
100g butternut squash, grated
50g butter, softened

*602 calories per portion
if serving 4; 401 if serving 6*

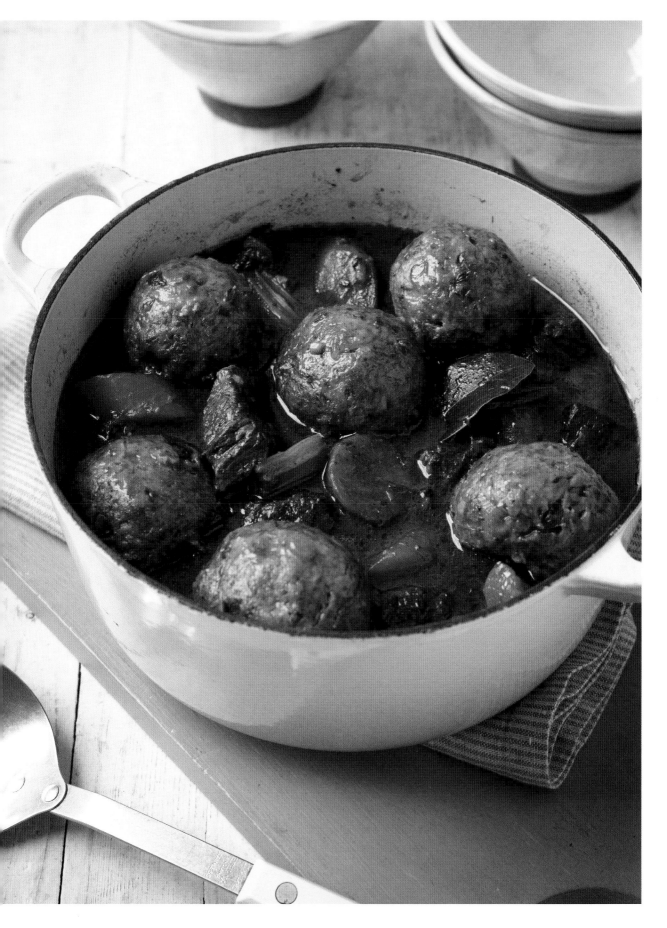

My Faves

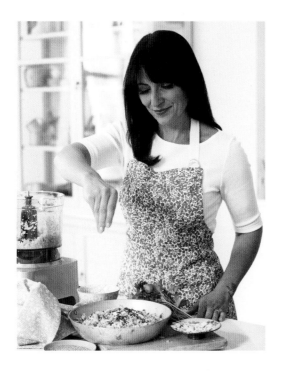

Chapter 6

Sides + Snacks

"Crisps were my weakness.
Not any more. Smart carbs rule."

Walnut and raisin bread

I never imagined myself making bread but you know what? It's a doddle and all that kneading is great exercise. Haha! I've even got you working out while you're cooking.

1 Put the flours, raisins, walnuts and yeast into a large bowl. Stir briefly, then add the salt and drizzle in the honey. Gradually add 300–350ml of lukewarm water to the bowl and mix to make a dough. Cover the bowl with a damp cloth or some cling film and leave the dough to rest for half an hour.

2 Turn the dough out on to a lightly floured surface and knead it until it's smooth – this will take about 10 minutes. Put the dough back in the bowl cover it again and leave it somewhere warm until it's doubled in size. It'll need at least a couple of hours.

3 Preheat the oven to its highest setting. Turn the dough out again and knead it lightly for a few moments. Shape the dough into an oval, making sure it is smooth and well rounded, then put it on a baking tray. Slash diagonal lines along the top with a serrated knife, then cover the loaf and leave it to stand for another 30–45 minutes.

4 Sprinkle the loaf with flour, then put it in the preheated oven and immediately turn the temperature down to 200°C/180°C Fan/Gas 6. Bake for 35–40 minutes, until the flour topping is a rich golden brown and the loaf sounds hollow when you tap it. Transfer the loaf to a wire rack and leave it to cool before slicing.

Makes 16 slices

200g wholemeal rye flour
300g wholemeal wheat flour, plus
  more for sprinkling
75g raisins, soaked in warm water
  for 5 minutes, then drained
75g walnuts, roughly chopped
7g instant dried yeast
300–350ml lukewarm water
7g salt
15g honey

161 calories per slice

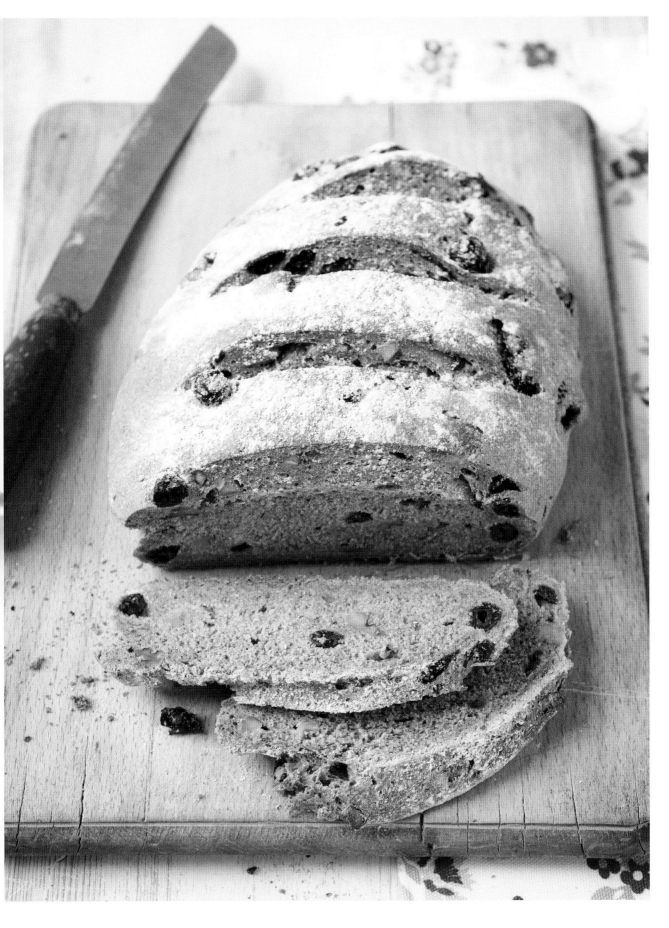

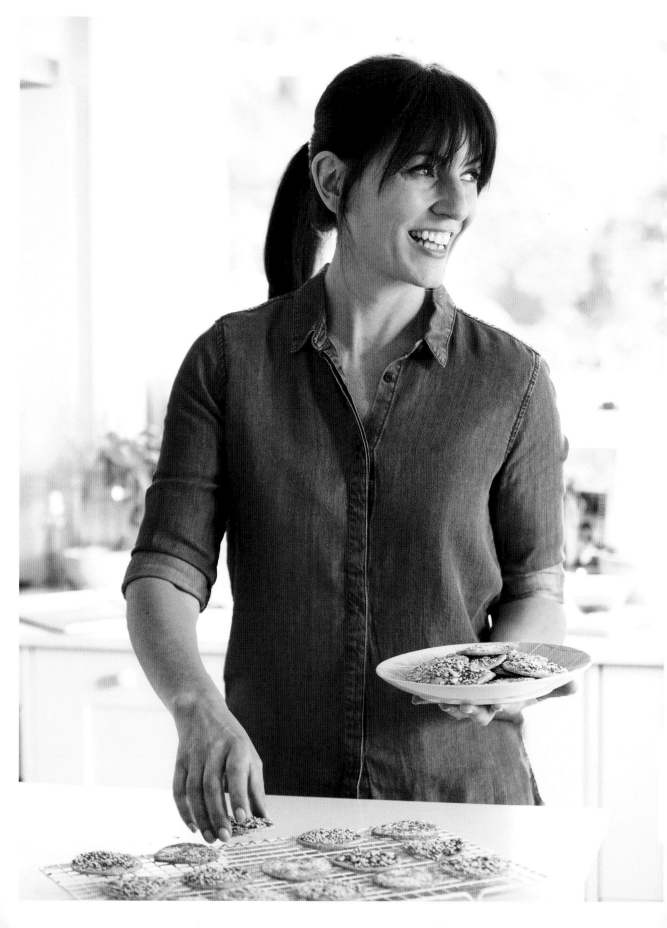

Spelt and rye crackers

Crispy crackers make a perfect snack with a dip or a sliver of cheese – and if you make your own you know exactly what's in them. I've suggested a couple of different toppings but you can have fun experimenting with your own flavours.

1 Preheat the oven to 180°C/160°C Fan/Gas 4. Mix the spelt and rye flours in a bowl and add the salt. Drizzle over the olive oil and stir it into the flour, then make a well in the middle. Gradually work in 125–150ml of water, stopping at 125ml to check if the dough clumps together properly. If it doesn't, add a little more water until you can form a ball that's not too crumbly.

2 Generously flour the work surface, then gently knead the dough until it's smooth. Roll it out until it's as thin as you can make it – this amount of dough should make a rectangle the size of a regular 20 x 30cm baking tray.

3 Cut the crackers into rounds with a 7cm diameter cookie cutter, or into any shape you like, and arrange them on a couple of baking trays.

4 Whisk the egg white with a tablespoon of water and brush it over the crackers. Sprinkle them with your choice of topping, then prick them all with a fork. Don't stint on this step or the crackers may puff up.

5 Bake the crackers in the preheated oven for 15–20 minutes, until they are crisp and golden. Make sure the undersides are completely dry. If you've topped your crackers with cheese they may need to cook for a little longer.

6 Remove the crackers from the oven and immediately transfer them to a rack. Once cool, they should have a good snap without any chewiness. Store the crackers in an airtight container.

Makes about 24

200g wholemeal spelt flour,
    plus extra for dusting
100g rye flour
½ tsp salt
1 tbsp olive oil
1 egg white

Topping
1 tbsp poppy seeds
1 tbsp sesame seeds
1 tbsp sunflower seeds
or
2 tbsp grated cheese
1 tbsp dried rosemary

61 calories per cracker with seed topping; 55 with cheese topping

Oatcakes

Using both porridge oats and oatmeal gives a nice coarse texture to these oatcakes, but you can use all oatmeal if you like. Good with a bowl of soup or a bit of cheese, or just whenever you feel like a crunchy mouthful.

1 Put the oatmeal and oats in a large bowl and mix in the salt. Put the butter in a separate bowl, then pour the water over it and stir until the butter has melted. Pour the butter and water mixture into the bowl of oats and mix briefly.

2 Clump the mixture together with your hands to make a fairly damp, but still crumbly dough. Wrap the dough in cling film and leave it to chill in the fridge for half an hour. Preheat the oven to 200°C/180°C Fan/Gas 6.

3 Roll the dough out on a floured surface until it is 2–3mm thick. Cut out rounds with a 7cm pastry cutter, re-rolling the dough when necessary. Using a palette knife, transfer the rounds to 2 baking trays.

4 Bake the oatcakes for 20–25 minutes, until they're browned around the edges and firm. Carefully transfer them to a wire rack and leave them to cool. Store the oatcakes in an airtight tin.

Makes about 20

200g medium oatmeal
100g porridge oats
½ tsp salt
100g butter, softened
100ml just-boiled water
flour, for dusting

96 calories per oatcake

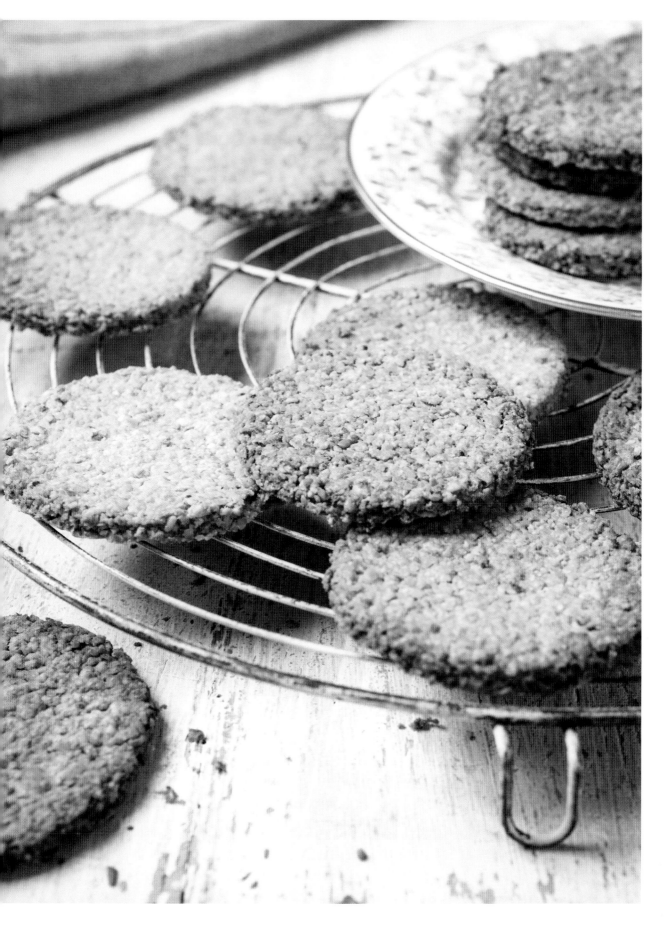

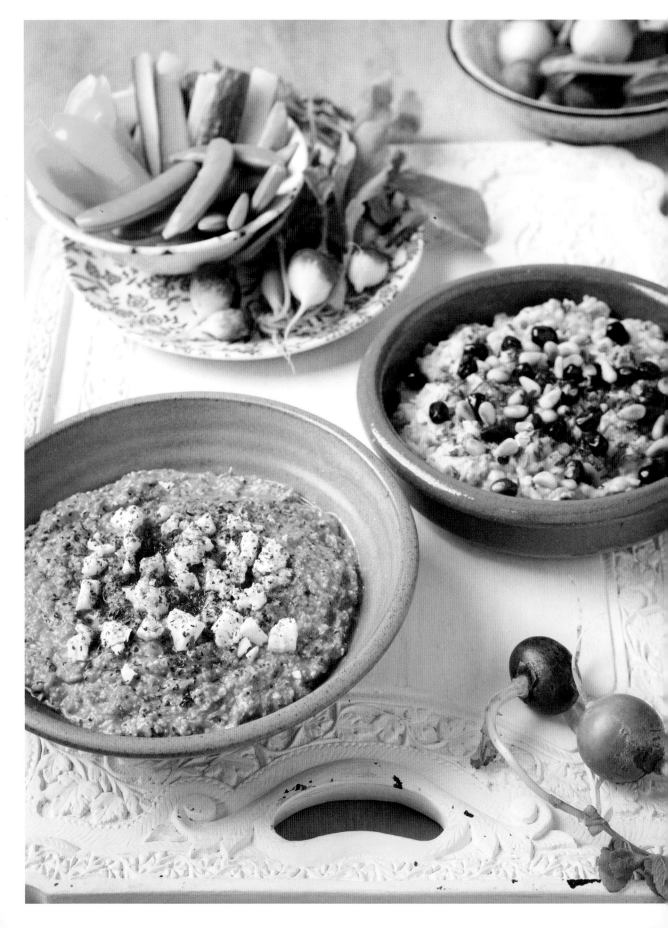

Dips

I love having a yummy dip in the fridge to dig into when the hunger pangs strike. Add some sticks of raw veg and you have an instant starter. The aubergine recipe is based on baba ganoush, a Middle Eastern classic. And the red pepper dip contains my favourite feta cheese.

Aubergine dip

1 Preheat the oven to 200°C/180°C Fan/Gas 6. Prick the aubergines all over with the tip of a sharp knife and place them on a baking tray. Roast the aubergines in the oven for about an hour, turning them occasionally, until they have started to blacken and collapse. Remove the aubergines from the oven and set them aside to cool slightly.

2 When the aubergines are cool enough to handle, peel them and put the flesh in a sieve or colander over the sink or a bowl. Sprinkle with salt and leave the flesh to drain for a few minutes to get rid of any excess liquid.

3 Roughly chop the aubergine flesh so it isn't too stringy, then put it in a bowl with the lemon juice, garlic, tahini and olive oil. Mix thoroughly. Taste to check the seasoning and add black pepper and more salt if necessary. Transfer the dip to a serving bowl and sprinkle with the pine nuts, if using, and the pomegranate seeds and herbs.

Makes about 14 x 30g servings

2 large aubergines (about 600g)
juice of 1 lemon
2 garlic cloves, crushed
1 tbsp tahini
1 tbsp olive oil
salt and black pepper

To garnish

15g pine nuts, lightly toasted (optional)
1 tbsp pomegranate seeds
1 tbsp mint, roughly chopped
1 tbsp coriander leaves or parsley

20 calories per serving

Roast red pepper and feta dip

1 Preheat the oven to 200°C/180°C Fan/Gas 6. Put the red peppers on a baking tray and roast them for 30–40 minutes until the skin has started to blacken and the flesh is softening. Transfer the peppers to a bowl, cover with cling film, then leave them to steam. When they are cool enough to handle, remove the skins. If you're using ready-roasted peppers, just remove them from the jar and drain off the liquid.

2 Put the flesh in a food processor or blender. Add the garlic and most of the feta, reserving about 20g to use as a garnish. Add the olive oil and blitz the mixture until it's fairly smooth, then transfer it to a serving bowl. Crumble over the reserved feta and drizzle over a little more olive oil. Sprinkle with dried mint and some cayenne.

Makes about 14 x 30g servings

3 red peppers, halved and deseeded or jar of ready-roasted red peppers
2 garlic cloves
200g feta cheese
1 tbsp olive oil, plus extra for drizzling
½ tsp dried mint
pinch of cayenne

34 calories per serving

Chickpea flatbreads

In the South of France they make brilliant flatbreads known as socca from chickpea flour. You cook them like pancakes and you can make large thin versions to use as wraps or smaller, thicker ones for scooping up dips. To use as flatbreads for scooping, make quite small thick pancakes – about 20cm in diameter. These also work well in my special lasagne (see page 94). For wraps, make your flatbreads larger and slightly thinner – roughly 26–28cm in diameter.

1 Sieve the chickpea flour into a large bowl. Add the salt, then gradually whisk in the water until you have a smooth, fairly thin batter. Leave the batter to stand for at least half an hour.

2 Spray a non-stick frying pan with olive oil and heat it over a medium-high flame. Ladle some of the batter into the pan and immediately swirl it around, making sure the batter spreads to the edges of the pan and completely covers the base. Cook on that side until the batter has set, then flip it over and cook on the other side. Remove the flatbread and keep it warm on a plate.

3 Spray the pan with oil again, add more batter and repeat. Continue until you have used up all the batter. The batter will keep in the fridge for several days if need be.

Makes 8 large or 12 smaller flatbreads (F)

300g chickpea (gram) flour
1 tsp salt
600ml water (room temperature)
olive oil spray

141 calories per large flatbread;
94 per smaller flatbread

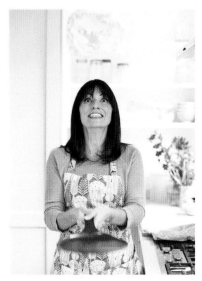
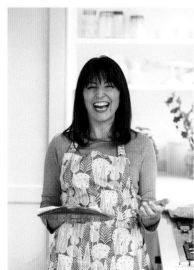

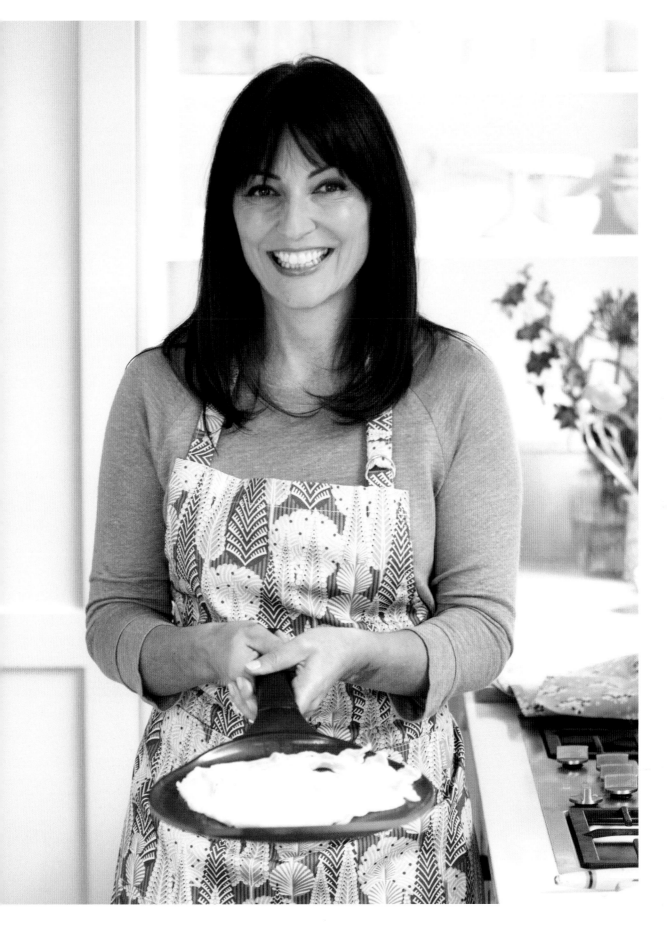

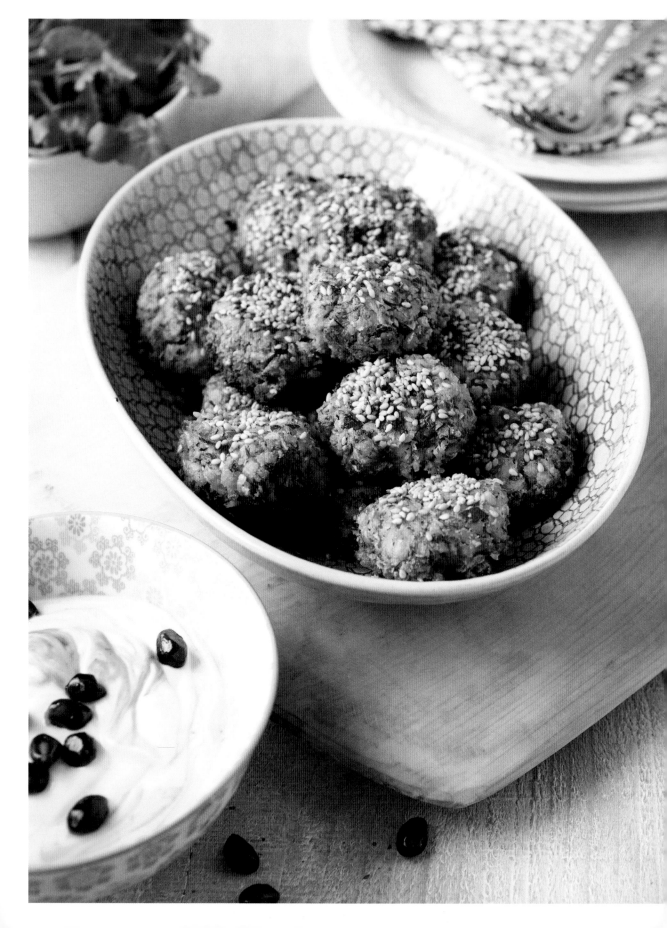

Broad bean falafel

Please don't tell anyone, but for some reason, Matthew's nickname for me is 'Falafel'. I know. In fact, I've always loved falafel and I've now discovered that they're easy to do and so much better than the ready-made versions, especially served with this yoghurt and pomegranate molasses dip. The pomegranate molasses is just pomegranate juice boiled to a fabulously sticky syrup and it has a sweet and sour flavour. You can buy it in supermarkets and you only need to use a small amount so it lasts for ages.

1 Put the broad beans, chickpeas and baking powder in a food processor and pulse to make a rough purée. Add the garlic, spring onions, lemon juice and zest, herbs and cumin, and season with salt and pepper. Be quite generous with the salt, as chickpeas can take quite a lot.

2 Transfer the mixture to a bowl and leave it in the fridge for half an hour to firm up. Preheat the oven to 220°C/200°C Fan/Gas 7.

3 Divide the mixture into 16 pieces and shape them into balls or little torpedo-shaped patties. Each ball should weigh 35–40g.

4 Put the olive oil and the sesame seeds in separate bowls. Dip your hands in the olive oil and pick up each falafel so it gets a coating of oil, then place it on a baking tray – you get a slightly more even result this way than by rolling the balls in the olive oil. Sprinkle the falafel with the sesame seeds. Bake the falafel in the preheated oven for 25–30 minutes until well browned and crisp.

5 Meanwhile, make the dip. Whisk together the yoghurt, pomegranate molasses and lemon juice and season with salt and pepper. Serve the falafel with the sauce for dipping.

Serves 4

250g broad beans, defrosted if frozen
250g cooked chickpeas
   (400g can, drained and rinsed, or
   freshly cooked – see p.205)
1 tsp baking powder
2 garlic cloves, finely chopped
4 spring onions, finely chopped
juice and zest of 1 lemon
small bunch of parsley, finely
   chopped
small bunch of mint, finely chopped
2 tbsp dill, finely chopped
½ tsp cumin
2 tbsp olive oil
25g sesame seeds
salt and black pepper

**Yoghurt and pomegranate
   molasses dip**
200ml Greek yoghurt
2 tbsp pomegranate molasses
1 tbsp lemon juice

292 calories per serving

Sweet potato fries

We all love chips if we're honest, and these are a healthier version that all the family will go crazy for. If you've invested in a vegetable spiraliser you can make cute little spirals of sweet potato. Otherwise, just cut them into chip shapes and they will taste just as good.

1 Peel the sweet potatoes and cut them into slender chips.

2 Soak the sweet potato chips in a bowl of iced water for half an hour, then drain them. This is important, as it removes the starch so the fries crisp up better. Dry them as thoroughly as you can – the easiest way to do this is to lay them out on a clean tea towel, then top with another tea towel and rub them gently. Preheat the oven to its highest setting.

3 Put the fries into a large bowl or bag and season them with salt and pepper. If using the spices, mix them with the flour. Add the flour to the fries and shake well to make sure they are all completely coated.

4 Lay the fries over 2 baking trays. Don't crowd them – they need plenty of room so they crisp up and don't steam. Drizzle them with the olive oil and toss gently, then bake them in the oven for about 20 minutes, turning them over half way through.

5 Remove the fries from the oven and serve them immediately.

Serves 4

500g sweet potatoes
½ tsp sweet smoked paprika (optional)
½ tsp garlic powder (optional)
½ tsp mustard powder (optional)
2 tbsp cornflour, rice flour or potato flour
2 tbsp olive oil
salt and black pepper

195 calories per serving

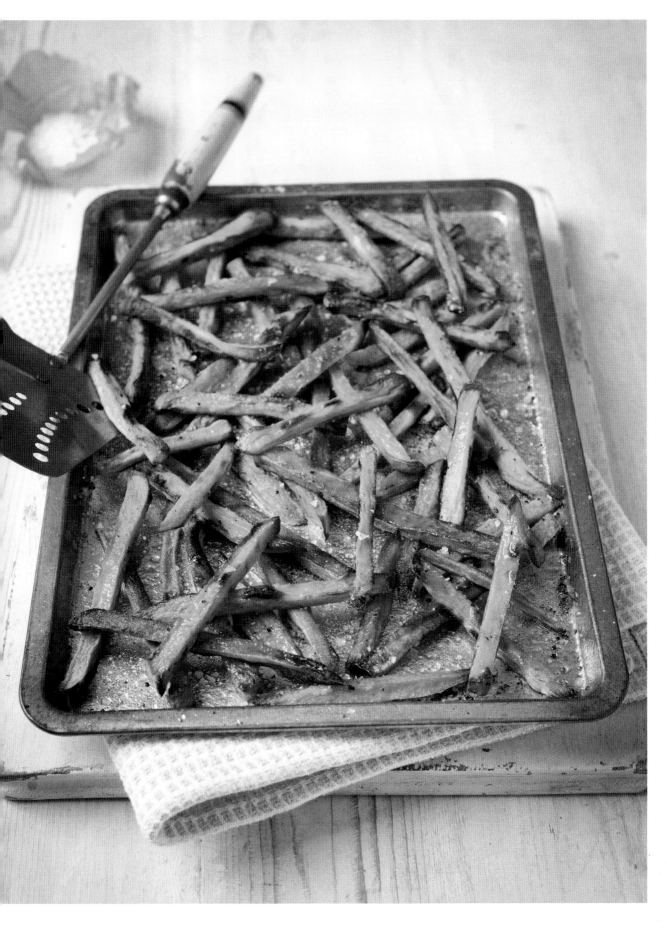

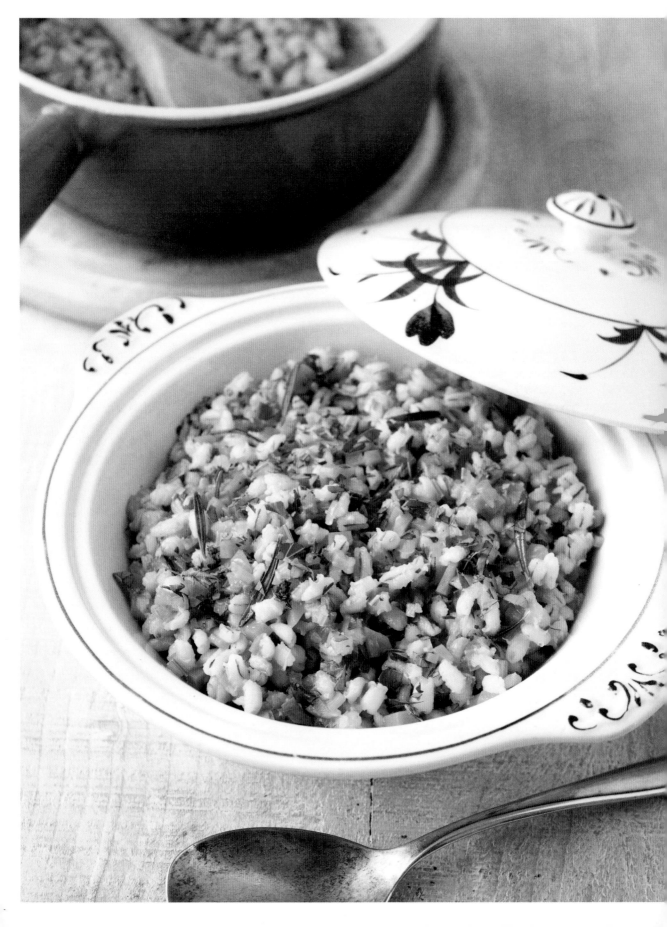

Braised barley

This is a really easy-going dish that you can enjoy on its own or serve with some cooked ham, grilled meat or just a salad. You could even add a bit of bacon to it – mmmm.

1 Heat the oil in a large saucepan or a casserole dish and add the onion, celery and carrot. Cook the vegetables for 5 minutes over a medium-high heat until they are starting to brown around the edges, stirring regularly.

2 Add the garlic, rosemary, lemon zest and barley. Stir for a couple of minutes, then pour the stock or water into the pan. Bring it to the boil, then turn down the heat and put a lid on the pan. Simmer the barley for 45–60 minutes, checking the liquid levels after the first half hour to make sure the pan isn't becoming too dry. Add a little more water or stock if necessary.

3 The barley is ready when it has absorbed the liquid but still has a little bite to it. Serve sprinkled with parsley.

Serves 4

1 tbsp olive oil
1 large onion, finely chopped
2 celery sticks, finely diced
1 large carrot (about 200g), diced
2 garlic cloves, finely chopped
1 large sprig of rosemary
zest of 1 lemon
250g pearl barley
1.5 litres chicken or vegetable stock
   or water
2 tbsp chopped parsley, to serve

347 calories per serving

Chickpea flour chips

This recipe is based on an amazing dish called panisse that's very popular in northern Italy and the South of France. The little chips are really light and fluffy and should be eaten straight away, as they lose their lightness quickly. Great on their own, dipped in mayonnaise or with a bit of chilli sauce. Yum, yum.

1 Lightly oil a 20 x 20cm baking tray and line it with cling film, making sure the cling film overlaps the sides.

2 Sift the flour into a saucepan and add a teaspoon of salt and lots of freshly ground pepper. Gradually whisk in 525ml of room temperature water, then put the pan over a low heat.

3 Stir the mixture over a low heat until it thickens to a dropping consistency. Pour the mixture into the baking tray and spread it out as evenly as possible. Leave for 20 minutes to set.

4 Slice the mixture into strips the size of fairly thin chips. You should get 35–40. Carefully remove them from the baking tray by lifting out the cling film.

5 Place a large frying pan over a medium-high heat and heat 2 tablespoons of the oil. Arrange half the chips in the frying pan and cook them on each of the long sides for a minute or so until they're golden brown. Drain them on kitchen paper, then repeat with the remaining oil and chips.

6 Serve the chips immediately, sprinkled with a little more salt and pepper and the herbs.

Serves 4

oil, for greasing
150g chickpea (gram) flour
525ml water (room temperature)
4 tbsp olive oil
1 tsp mixed dried herbs
salt and black pepper

240 calories per serving

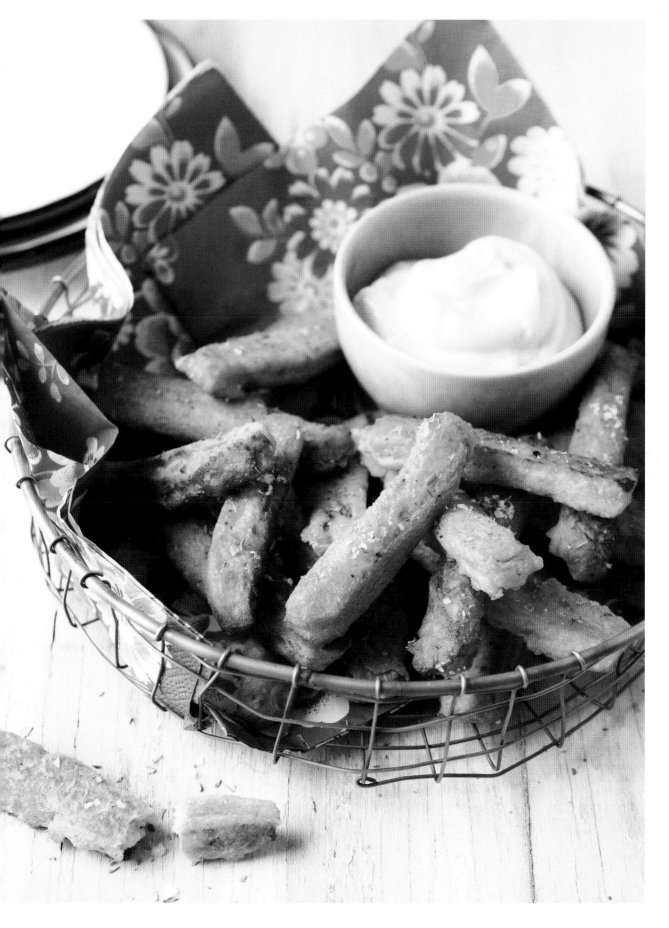

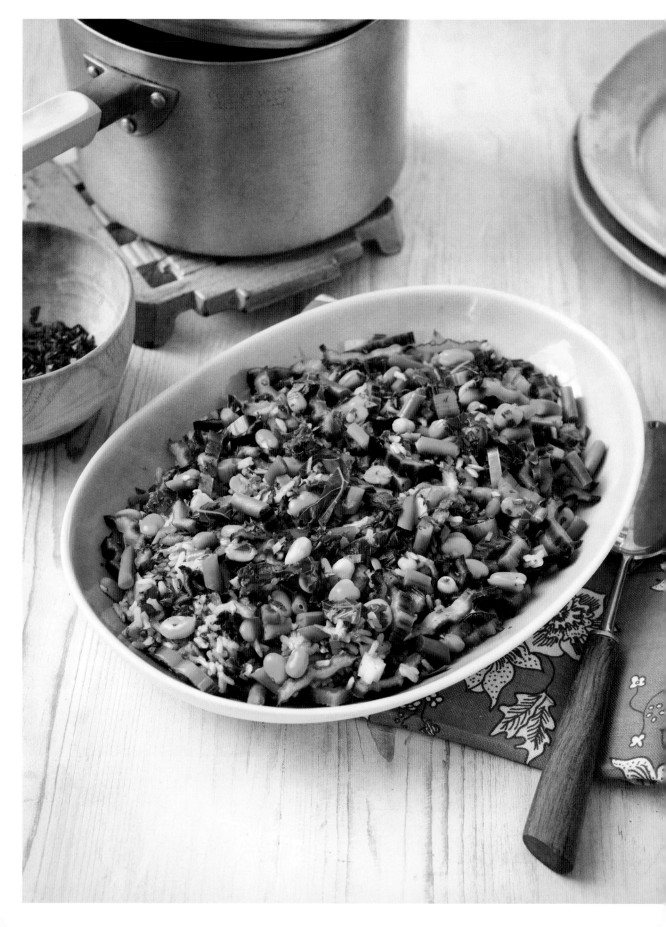

Brown rice pilaf

I love this clever way of bulking out a small amount of rice with lots of gorgeous green veg. It gives you a feeling of plenty without lots of calories. You could also make it with broccoli, sprouting broccoli or peas.

1 Soak the rice for 15 minutes in plenty of cold water, then drain it thoroughly. Heat the olive oil in a large saucepan, add the onion and cook it gently over a medium heat for a few minutes until it's starting to soften and brown.

2 Add the garlic, allspice, coriander and parsley stems and the lemon zest. Stir for a couple of minutes, then add the rice and cook for another 2 minutes. Pour the stock into the pan and season with salt and pepper.

3 Bring the stock to the boil, then cover the pan and cook the rice over a fairly high heat for 5 minutes. Remove the lid and add the broad beans, green beans and kale, cabbage or chard on top of the rice and liquid but don't stir them in. Put the lid back on the pan, turn down the heat and simmer for about 30 minutes or until the rice is tender.

4 Remove the pan from the heat and leave the rice and veg to stand for another 10 minutes. Don't remove the lid at this time or the steam will escape and stop the cooking process. Then stir the vegetables into the rice together with the herbs – the liquid should all have been absorbed and the vegetables should be tender.

5 Serve the pilaf immediately, either in the pot or on a serving dish, with a little lemon juice squeezed over it, if you like.

**Serves 6
as a side dish**

175g brown rice
1 tbsp olive oil
1 large onion, finely diced
2 garlic cloves, finely chopped
½ tsp ground allspice
small bunch of coriander, stems and
    leaves separated, finely chopped
small bunch of parsley, stems and
    leaves separated, finely chopped
zest of 1 lemon
400ml vegetable or chicken stock
200g broad beans, defrosted if frozen
100g green beans, cut into short
    rounds
150g kale, cabbage or chard, finely
    shredded
squeeze of lemon juice (optional)
salt and black pepper

186 calories per serving

Vegetable couscous

This makes an amazing low-carb, low-cal side dish. And if you add extras such as herbs and almonds it tastes even better. You can vary the herbs and spices to go with whatever you're eating.

1 Put the cauliflower and/or broccoli florets in a food processor and blitz them until they resemble breadcrumbs.

2 Heat the olive oil in a large, heavy-based frying pan. If you're using any spices, add these now and toast them in the oil for 30 seconds. Add the cauliflower and/or broccoli and stir everything together for a minute or so, then season with salt and pepper.

3 Pour 100ml of water into the pan and cook the veg over a medium heat for at least 5 minutes, stirring very frequently. By this time, the water should have all been absorbed and the 'couscous' should be dry with a little bite to it, without having a raw texture.

4 Remove the pan from the heat and fluff up the 'couscous' with a fork. Stir through extra herbs if you like and sprinkle with flaked almonds.

Serves 4

1 head of cauliflower, broken into
   florets or 600g broccoli florets
   or a combination
1 tbsp olive oil
salt and black pepper

Optional extras
whole spices, such as nigella or
   mustard seeds
chopped fresh herbs
flaked almonds, lightly toasted

76 calories per serving

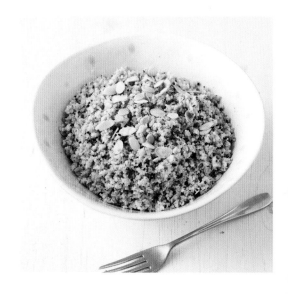

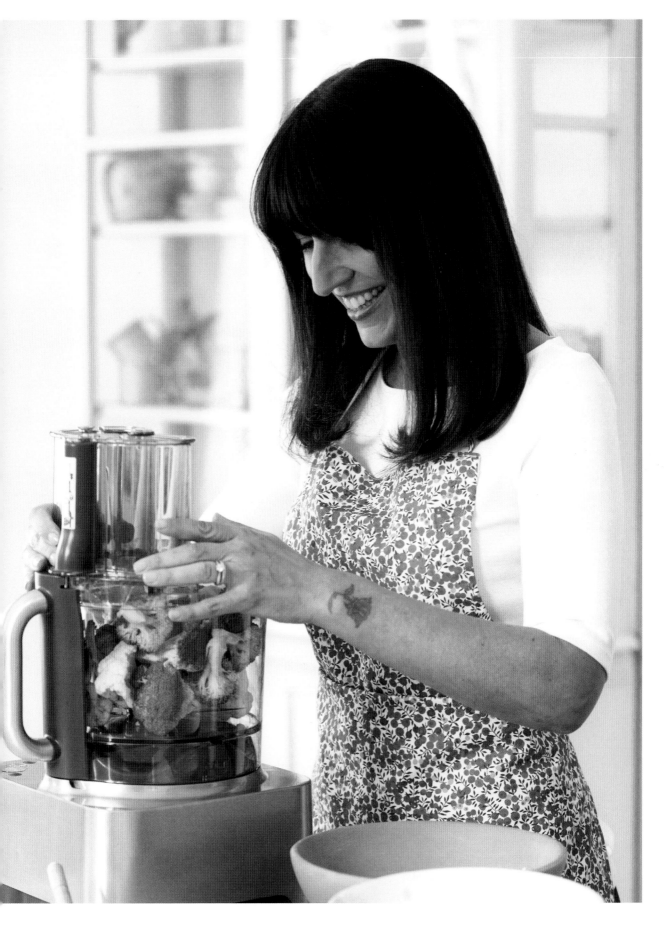

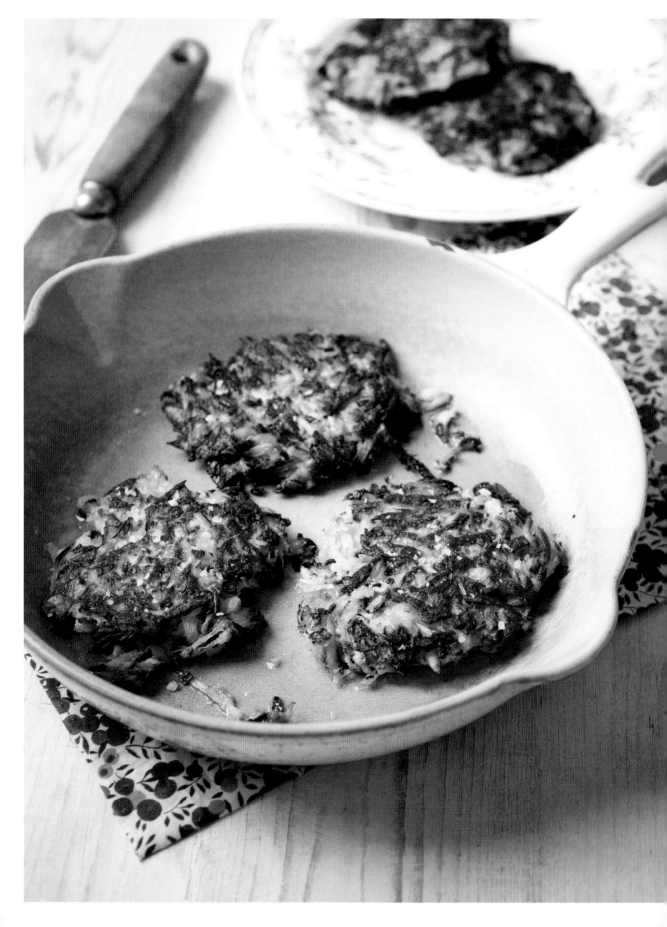

Parsnip rösti

I love rösti but I wanted to try making it with something other than white potatoes. This parsnip version works well, but you do need to squish the mixture together thoroughly and allow plenty of room in the frying pan so you can flip them over easily. Parsnips can be quite tricky to grate by hand so it's best to use a food processor if you have one.

1 Squeeze the grated parsnip over the sink to get rid of as much excess liquid as you can, then mix it with the onion, apple and sage in a bowl. Beat the egg lightly and add it to the bowl. Season with salt and pepper, then mix thoroughly to ensure the egg coats everything well.

2 Heat the olive oil in a very large frying pan. Form the parsnip mixture into 8 small patties and arrange them in the frying pan, making sure they are well spaced out. If you don't have a big pan, fry the rösti in a couple of batches. Cook the rösti over a medium heat for several minutes on each side, until they are a deep golden brown. This will probably take about 5 minutes on the first side, 3–4 minutes on the second.

3 Serve immediately with grilled meat, salad or whatever you fancy.

Serves 4

200g parsnips, coarsely grated
1 small onion, finely chopped
1 small eating apple, grated
½ tsp dried sage, thyme or rosemary
1 egg
1 tbsp olive oil
salt and black pepper

107 calories per serving

Popcorn

We're obsessed with popcorn in my household and thankfully it's far better for you than crisps, particularly if you make it at home so you can control what you put with it. Try these flavours, then experiment with some of your own and let me know how you're doing on FB or Twitter.

1 Heat a large saucepan, preferably one with a glass lid, over a medium heat. Add the oil and heat it for a minute, then add the popping corn. Swirl the corn a little so it's completely coated in oil, then put the lid on the pan and turn the heat down to low.

2 When you can hear the corn popping, hold the lid in place and wait until the corn stops hitting it – this can take longer than you think. When there are a few seconds in between each pop, remove the lid. Discard any unpopped kernels – there shouldn't be many – and add your chosen flavouring.

Serves 6

2 tsp vegetable oil
100g popping corn

75 calories per serving
(all the savoury recipes)

Mediterranean popcorn

Blitz the salt with the pepper, herbs and lemon zest to a fairly fine powder. Sprinkle this over the still warm popcorn and mix thoroughly.

1 tsp sea salt
½ tsp freshly ground black pepper
1 tsp herbes de Provence
zest of ½ lemon

Japanese popcorn

Break up the nori seaweed, then blitz it with the cayenne, a grinding of black pepper and a pinch of salt. Sprinkle this over the popcorn and mix thoroughly, then add a dash of soy sauce if you like.

2 sheets of nori seaweed
¼ tsp cayenne
a dash of light soy sauce or tamari
   (optional)
salt and black pepper

Salt and vinegar popcorn

Sprinkle the sea salt over warm popcorn and drizzle over the vinegar. Toss and serve immediately.

1 tsp sea salt
a few dashes of cider vinegar

Sweet popcorn

Gently heat the maple syrup with the lime zest, spices and a pinch of salt. Pour this over the popcorn and mix thoroughly.

2 tbsp maple syrup
zest of ½ lime
¼ tsp cinnamon
grating of nutmeg
pinch of salt

92 calories per serving

Smoky almonds

You can buy smoked salt in supermarkets, but don't worry too much if you can't get any – the smokiness of the paprika still gives a good flavour.

1 Heat the olive oil in a frying pan over a medium heat. Add the almonds and fry them for about 5 minutes until you can smell their lovely aroma, shaking the pan or stirring the nuts regularly.

2 Tip the almonds into a bowl, then sprinkle over the salt and paprika. Stir to combine, then store the almonds in an airtight container.

Makes 10 x 20g servings

1 tbsp olive oil
200g whole almonds, preferably with the skin on
½ tsp smoked sea salt, crushed
½ tsp sweet smoked paprika

142 calories per serving

Roasted chickpeas

A perfect spicy snack. Sumac is a spice with a lovely lemony tang and it's popular in Middle Eastern cooking. You can find it in the supermarket, but just leave it out if you don't have any.

1 Preheat the oven to 220°C/200°C Fan/Gas 7. Put the chickpeas in a bowl and drizzle the oil over them. Mix the herbs, lemon zest, cayenne and sumac with a teaspoon of salt and plenty of freshly ground black pepper. Sprinkle this over the chickpeas and mix thoroughly.

2 Spread the chickpeas over a baking tray. Roast them in the oven for 30–40 minutes, checking them regularly and giving the tray a shake from time to time so the chickpeas roast evenly.

3 When the chickpeas are crisp and have a crunchy texture, remove them from the oven and leave them to cool. Add a little more sumac if you like, then transfer the chickpeas to an airtight container.

Makes 5 x 50g portions

400 can of chickpeas, drained and rinsed, or 240–250g cooked chickpeas (see p.205)
1 tbsp olive oil
1 tsp mixed herbs
1 tsp lemon zest
½ tsp cayenne
1 tsp sumac (optional)
salt and black pepper

71 calories per serving

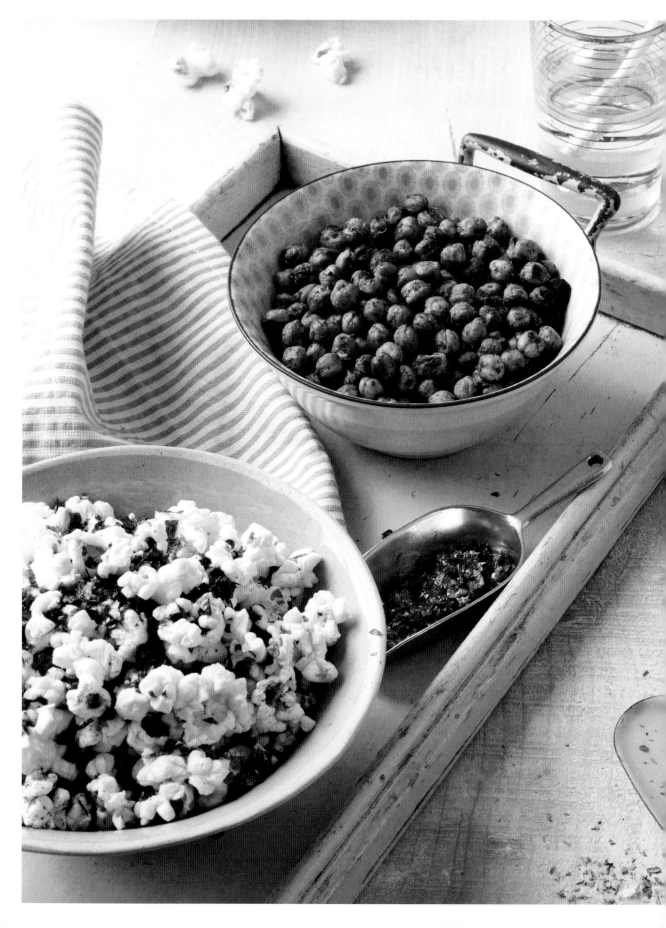

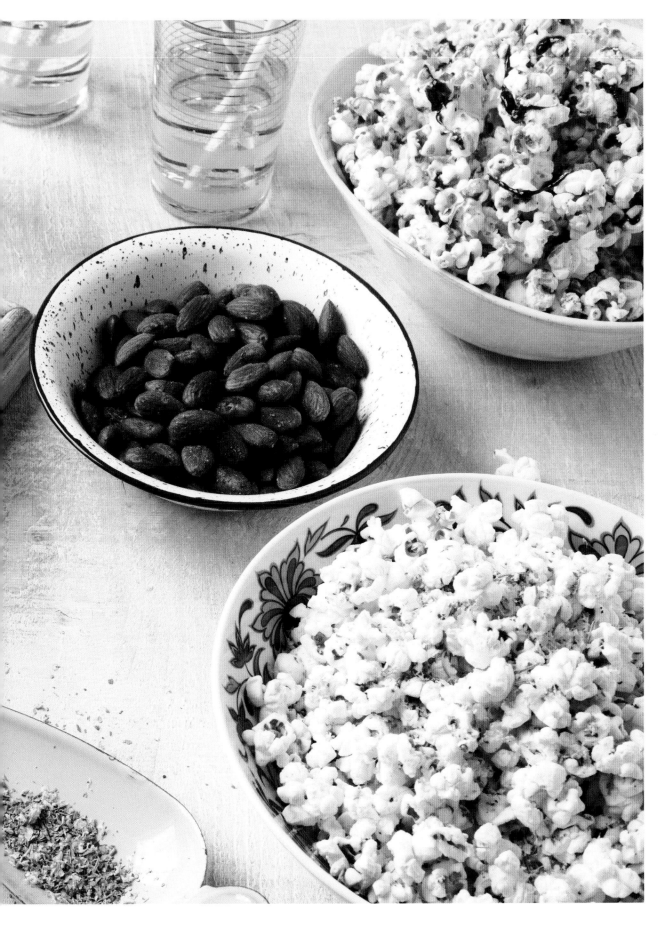

Apricot and pistachio power balls

Everyone loved the power balls in 5 *Weeks to Sugar Free* so we just had to come up with a new version – these are fruity and fabulous. I like the touch of maple syrup, but you can leave it out if you prefer. And you can add a little spice – such as cinnamon, ground ginger or cardamom. If you don't have any pistachios, use almonds instead.

1 Put the apricots in a food processor and pulse until they are very finely chopped. Add the remaining ingredients and process until the mixture comes together.

2 Roll the mixture into balls the size of a walnut. Put the ground or finely chopped pistachios on a plate and roll the balls in them until they're completely coated. Chill the balls until they're firm and store them in an airtight container in the fridge.

Makes about 16

150g dried apricots
100g nut butter, preferably
 unsalted
50g desiccated coconut or
 oatmeal
50g pistachios, finely chopped
1 tbsp maple syrup (optional)

For rolling
25g pistachios, finely chopped or
 ground

106 calories per power ball

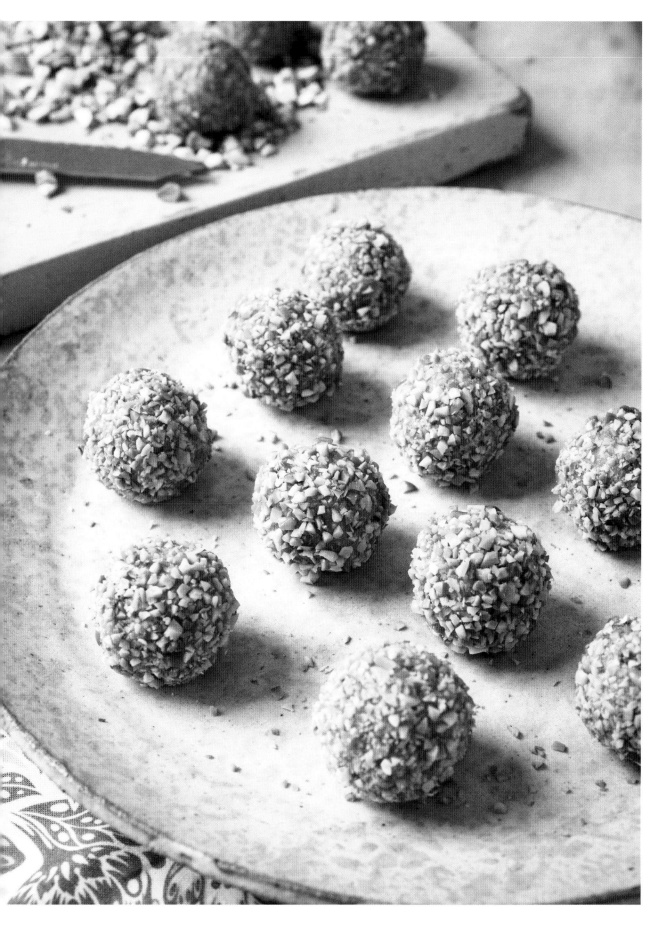

My Faves

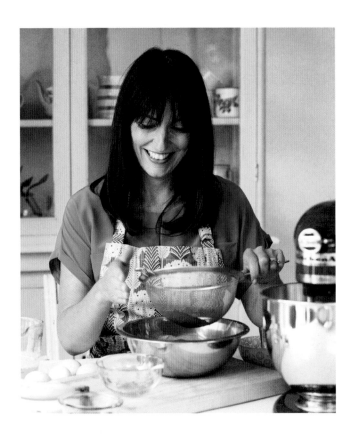

Chapter 7

Cakes + Puddings

"In true life (as my kids used to say),
we all need a treat every now and then.
These beauties – all free from refined
sugar – will satisfy your sweet tooth
without ruining your waistline. Yum."

Baked plums

Plums go beautifully with a little hint of spice. This is quick to make and hugely popular with all my family. The cardamom seeds add a fragrant flavour, but if you don't have any, the plums still taste good without them.

1 Preheat the oven to 200°C/180°C Fan/Gas 6. Grease an ovenproof dish with a little butter. Place the plums, cut side up, in the dish.

2 Put the 25g of honey with the butter in a small saucepan and warm them over a gentle heat until they've melted together. Remove the saucepan from the heat and stir the almonds and spices into the butter and honey. The mixture should be quite crumbly, but it should clump together when squeezed.

3 Spoon about a dessertspoon of the mixture into the centre of each plum half. Bake the plums in the oven for about 15 minutes or until they have completely softened and the topping is golden brown.

4 Whisk the honey, if using, into the crème fraiche or yoghurt. Serve the plums with dollops of the sweetened crème fraiche and a few more flaked almonds as a garnish, if you like.

Serves 4

25g butter, plus extra for greasing
8 ripe plums, halved and stones
  removed
25g honey
75g ground almonds
25g flaked almonds, plus extra
  to garnish
seeds from 3 cardamom pods,
  ground
¼ tsp ground ginger
pinch of cinnamon

To serve
1 tbsp honey (optional)
150g crème fraiche or yoghurt

414 calories per serving

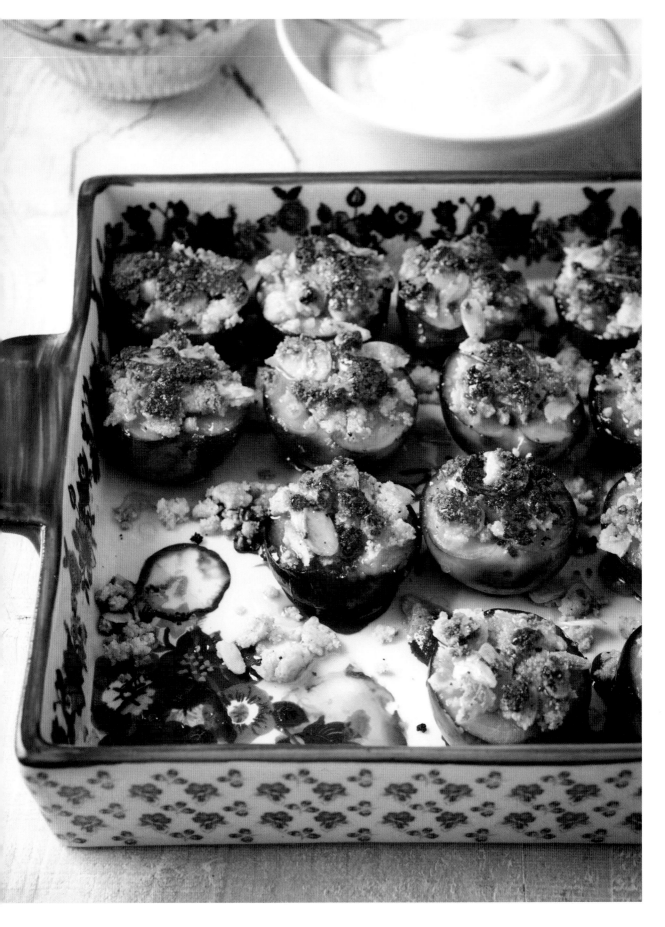

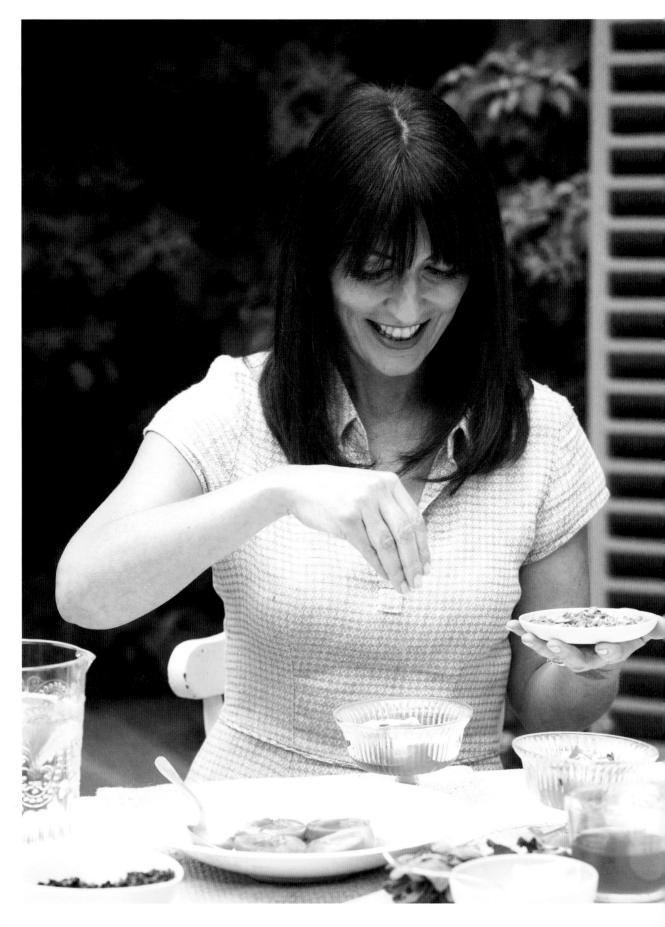

Poached peaches with pistachios

Make this in the summer when peaches are at their luscious best. You may or may not need the extra honey for serving, depending on how sweet your fruit is, so see what you think. Really pretty – just like you.

1 Select a saucepan that's just large enough to hold the peaches snugly. Put the 100 grams of honey in the pan with 500ml of water and slowly bring to the boil, stirring until the honey has dissolved.

2 Add the rose water, then put the peaches into the pan, cut-side up. You should find the liquid comes just up to the top of them. Cover the pan and simmer the peaches for 5–10 minutes, depending on how ripe they are. Keep an eye on the peaches, as you want them to keep their shape and not fall apart.

3 Remove the saucepan from the heat and leave the peaches to cool in the honey water. As soon as they are cool enough to handle, peel off any remaining skin – you should find most of it has slipped off during cooking. Put the peaches back in the saucepan and set them aside to cool completely.

4 Serve the peaches with a dollop of crème fraiche and a teaspoon of extra honey per person if you want extra sweetness, then sprinkle over some chopped pistachios or mint leaves and the rose petals. Wait for the gasps of admiration.

Serves 4

4 ripe but firm peaches,
   cut in half and stones removed
100g honey
1 tsp rose water

To serve
4 dsrtsp crème fraiche
4 tsp honey (optional)
chopped pistachios or
   mint leaves
dried rose petals

200 calories per serving

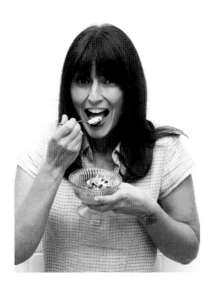

Chocolate panna cotta

OMG . . . this is so good. We've made it with dark, dark chocolate and as little sweetness as poss and it is incredible, I promise. Don't be tempted to cut down on the cream, or the recipe won't work as well. I used to avoid anything with gelatine or vanilla pods, but then I used both in *5 Weeks to Sugar Free* and now I'm a dab hand. There's nothing to be scared of. Trust me . . . I'm a presenter.

1 Brush 4 ramekins with vegetable oil and wipe off any excess with kitchen paper. Put the gelatine leaves in a small dish, cover them with cold water and leave them to soak for 5 minutes until softened.

2 In a small bowl, whisk 2 tablespoons of the milk with the cocoa powder and set it aside. Pour the remaining milk and the double cream into a saucepan, add the chocolate, honey and vanilla seeds and heat until the chocolate and honey have melted.

3 Remove the pan from the heat. Pour some of the heated mixture over the cocoa and milk mixture, then pour it all back into the saucepan and whisk to mix thoroughly. Wring out the excess water from the gelatine sheets and add them to the saucepan. Put the pan over a gentle heat and stir until the gelatine has dissolved. Don't let the mixture boil.

4 Pour the mixture through a sieve into a jug, then divide it between the ramekins. Cover the panna cottas with cling film and leave them to cool, then put them in the fridge for several hours until they have set completely.

5 To serve, dip the ramekins into just-boiled water for a few seconds to loosen the panna cottas, then turn them out on to plates.

Serves 4

vegetable oil, for greasing
3 leaves of gelatine
250ml whole milk
1 tbsp cocoa powder
200ml double cream
30g dark chocolate
    (100% cocoa solids, if possible)
100g honey
seeds scraped from ½ split
    vanilla pod

418 calories per serving

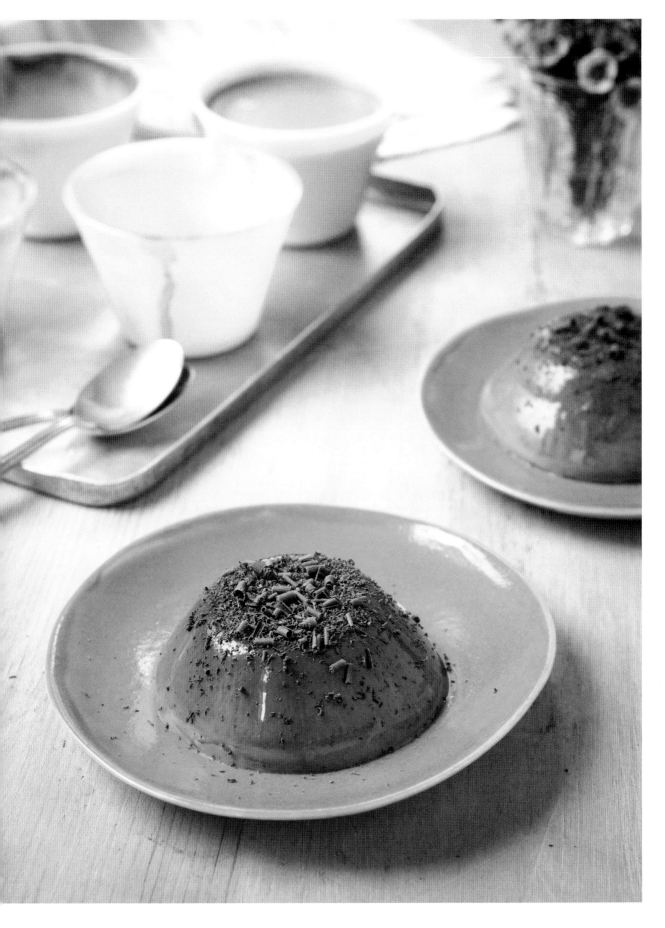

Frozen yoghurt

This is lovely just as it is or you could stir in some chopped strawberries or raspberries when churning.

1 Put the yoghurt in a bowl with the maple syrup or honey. Squeeze in the lime juice and add a small pinch of salt, then whisk until everything is well combined.

2 If you're using an ice cream maker, churn the yoghurt mixture until it's the consistency of ice cream. Scrape it all into a tub and freeze immediately. If not using an ice cream maker, put the yoghurt into a large tub, freeze it for an hour, then whisk. Repeat the freezing and whisking a couple of times – this will help the yoghurt incorporate air and make it softer.

3 Remove the yoghurt from the freezer 5 minutes before serving so it has a chance to soften to a scoopable texture.

Serves 4

500ml thick Greek yoghurt
75ml maple syrup or honey
juice of half a lime
salt

214 calories per serving

Watermelon and cherry slush

Wonderfully refreshing on a hot day, this is a version of granita but much softer and slushier. Incredibly easy to make.

1 Put all the ingredients in a blender and blitz until the mixture is as smooth as possible. Push the mixture through a sieve to get rid of anything too fibrous, then pour it into a shallow plastic container.

2 Put it in the freezer and freeze until solid, then blitz to a slush when you're ready to serve. Or, if you're in a rush, it's fine just to freeze the mixture until it's semi-frozen, then blitz to serve. Nice scooped into little glasses or ramekins.

Serves 4

250g cherries, pitted
300g watermelon, peeled and deseeded
juice of 2 limes
75g honey

110 calories per serving

Jellies

Lots of people get nervous about using gelatine. I used to get nervous about using gelatine, but I'm proud to say I have conquered my fear. Just soak it, squeeze it and you're away. Different brands do vary slightly in size and strength, so check the packet for the recommended number of sheets per 100ml of liquid and you'll be fine.

Coconut water jelly

1 Put the coconut water in a saucepan and add a squeeze of lime juice. Heat gently until the liquid is finger hot, but not boiling. Wring out the gelatine and add it to the coconut water. Stir until it has completely dissolved, making sure you keep the mixture over a low temperature.

2 Strain the liquid into a jelly mould or 4 individual moulds. Allow it to cool, then add the berries. Stir regularly until the jelly has begun to thicken, just to make sure the fruit doesn't all sink to the bottom. Transfer the jelly to the fridge to set. Serve well chilled.

Serves 4

500ml coconut water
squeeze of lime juice
4–5 gelatine leaves, soaked
   in cold water for 5 minutes
150g blueberries and/or raspberries

47 calories per serving

Orange and lime juice jelly

1 Put the orange juice and lime juice in a saucepan with the honey, if using. Heat through, stirring, until the honey has dissolved. Wring out the gelatine and add it to the juice.

2 Stir until the gelatine has completely dissolved, then strain the liquid into a big jelly mould or individual jelly moulds. Leave to cool, then transfer the jelly to the fridge to set. Serve well chilled.

Serves 4

500ml freshly squeezed orange juice
   (about 6 large oranges)
juice of 1 lime
1 tbsp honey (optional)
4–5 leaves of gelatine, soaked in cold
   water for 5 minutes

47 calories per serving

Fruits of the forest jelly

1 Put the frozen fruit in a saucepan and add 200ml of the fruit juice. Simmer gently until the fruit looks swollen and very juicy. Allow the mixture to cool slightly, then transfer it to a blender and blitz until smooth as possible. Push it through a sieve.

2 Measure the puréed liquid and make it up to 700ml with the extra juice. Pour it back into the pan and add the honey, if using. Reheat, then wring out the gelatine, add it to the liquid and stir until completely dissolved. Strain the mixture into a jelly mould or individual moulds and leave it to cool. Transfer it to the fridge to set and serve chilled.

Serves 4

500g pack frozen fruits of the forest
up to 300ml fruit juice – grape, apple,
   pear, cherry are all good
1 tbsp honey (optional)
8 leaves gelatine, soaked in cold
   water for 5 minutes

71 calories per serving

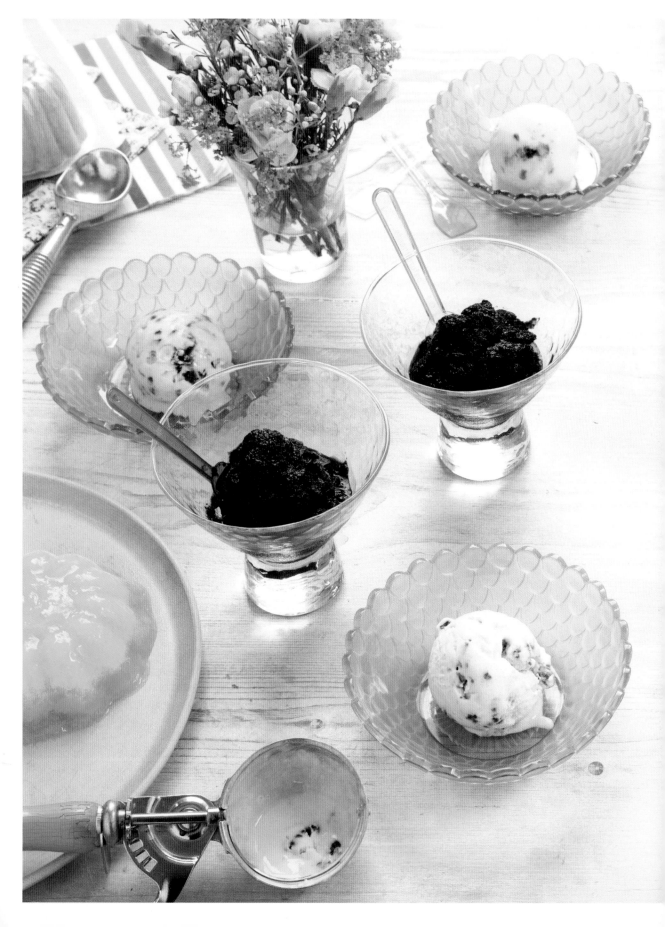

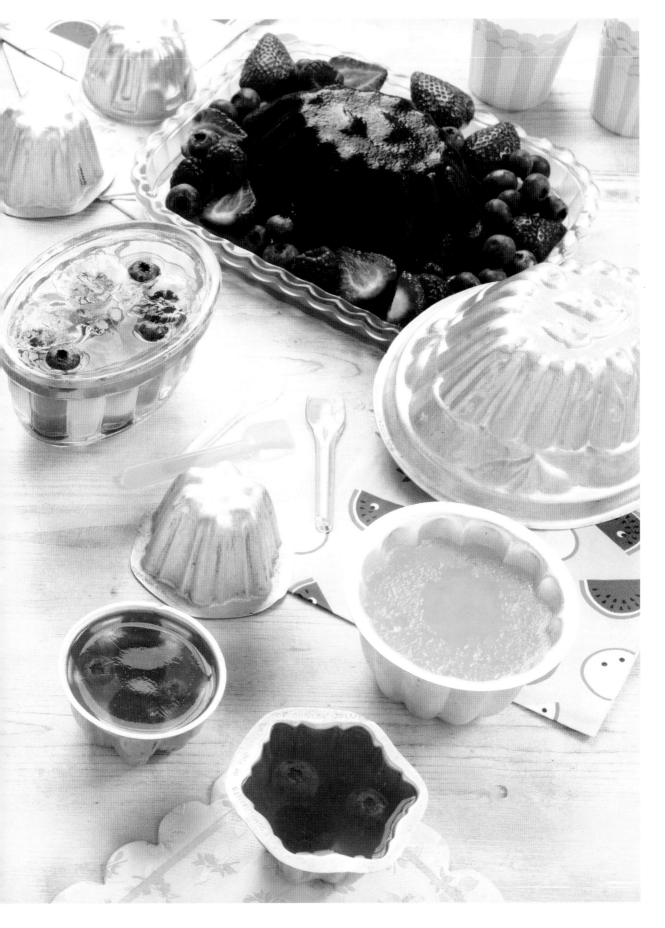

Sticky toffee pudding

Matthew and I had this at our wedding and I love, love, love it. There's no such thing as a completely guilt-free sticky toffee pudding, but hey – this is an occasional treat. I have to admit that the sauce is high-cal so you could leave it to the non-dieters and just have the sponge with some Greek yoghurt. Over to you.

1 Preheat the oven to 180°C/160°C Fan/Gas 4. Grease a square baking tin or an ovenproof dish with butter, then dust it with flour.

2 Put the dates in a bowl with the bicarbonate of soda and 300ml of just-boiled water. Leave the dates to steep, breaking them up with a wooden spoon as they begin to soften, until you can stir them into a fairly smooth paste. If necessary, blitz the dates in a food processor for a few seconds.

3 Put the flour and baking powder in a large bowl with a pinch of salt and whisk thoroughly to combine and to break up any lumps.

4 Add the maple syrup, butter, eggs and the seeds from the vanilla pod to the dates, then add this mixture to the flour. Stir until you have a smooth batter.

5 Spoon the batter into the prepared baking tin or dish. Bake the pudding in the oven for 35–40 minutes, until the sponge is firm and springy to touch and is shrinking away from the sides.

6 To make the sauce, put the butter and maple syrup in a saucepan with the seeds from the vanilla pod and a pinch of salt. Simmer over a low heat until the butter has melted, then add half the cream. Turn up the heat slightly and whisk to combine for 3–4 minutes, then add the rest of the cream. Serve piping hot with the pud.

Serves 8

butter, for greasing
flour, for dusting
200g pitted dates, chopped
½ tsp bicarbonate of soda
300ml just-boiled water
175g wholemeal flour or
  wholemeal spelt flour
1 tsp baking powder
pinch of salt
125ml maple syrup
50g butter, softened
2 eggs, beaten
seeds scraped from ½ vanilla pod

Sauce
50g butter
100ml maple syrup
seeds scraped from ½ vanilla pod
pinch of salt
200ml single cream

345 calories per serving
with sauce; 218 without sauce

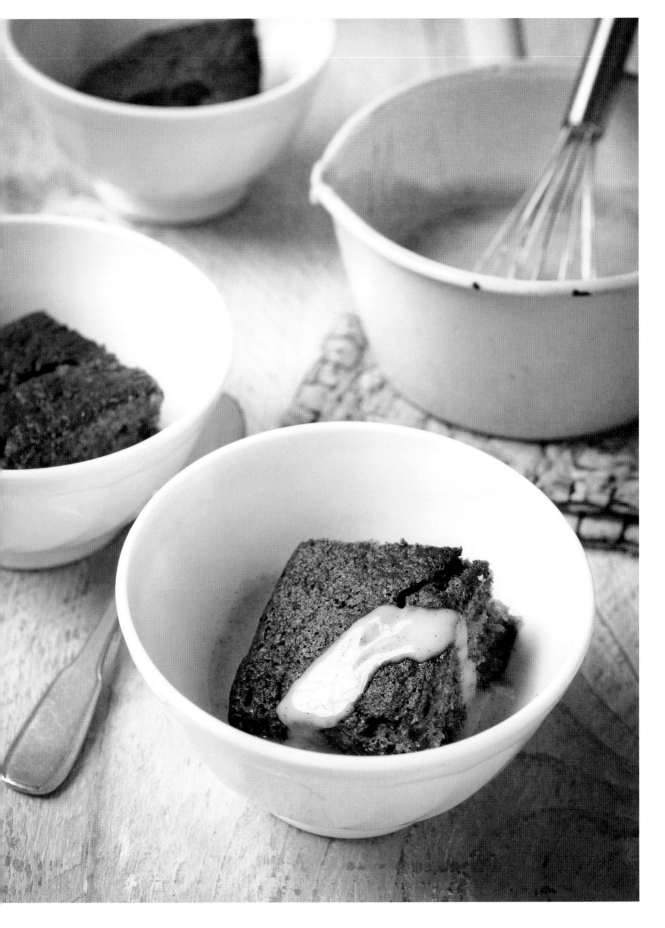

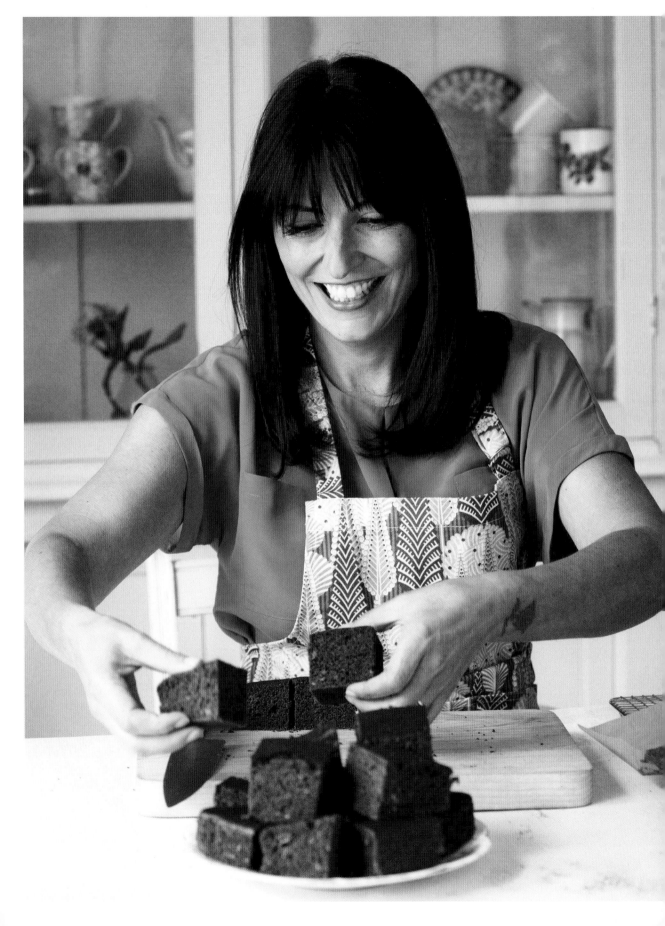

Chocolate and banana tray bake

Eaten while it's still slightly warm from the oven, this is beyond amazing. Yes, there are a lot of eggs in it but they are what make the cake lovely and light. And yes, there's maple syrup so quite a few calories, but you're only going to eat one square – aren't you?

1 Preheat the oven to 180°C/160°C Fan/Gas 4. Line a 24 x 24cm tray bake tin with baking parchment.

2 Sift the flour, cocoa and baking powder into a bowl and add a pinch of salt. Put the butter in a small pan and melt it over a gentle heat. Remove the pan from the heat, stir in the maple syrup, then mix in the mashed bananas.

3 Break the eggs into a large bowl and whisk them until they're frothy. Add the dry ingredients, then the butter, syrup and banana mixture and mix thoroughly. Pour the mixture into the prepared tin and spread it into an even layer.

4 Bake the cake in the oven for about 40 minutes until it's well risen, springy to touch and shrinking away from the sides slightly. Leave it to cool in the tin for 10 minutes, then transfer it to a cooling rack. Cut it into 16 squares – or smaller pieces if you want to reduce the calorie count per serving. Store the cake in an airtight tin.

Makes 16 squares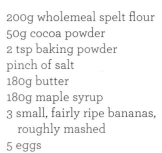

200g wholemeal spelt flour
50g cocoa powder
2 tsp baking powder
pinch of salt
180g butter
180g maple syrup
3 small, fairly ripe bananas, roughly mashed
5 eggs

212 calories per square

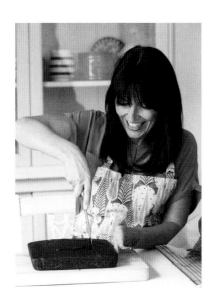

Orange and almond cake

There's no flour in this cake – just ground almonds – so it is quite dense but still lovely and moist. It's perfect served just as it is with a cup of tea or as a pud with yoghurt or crème fraiche. If you like, you can cook the oranges the night before so they have time to cool down, all ready for you to make the cake the next day.

1 Put the oranges in a saucepan and cover them with water. Bring the water to the boil, then put a lid on the pan and simmer the oranges for 1–1½ hours until they're very soft. You should be able to pierce the skin easily with the handle of a wooden spoon.

2 Drain the oranges and set them aside to cool. When they're cool enough to handle, cut them in half and remove any pips. Put the oranges in a food processor and blitz them to a purée.

3 Preheat the oven to 180°C/160°C Fan/Gas 4. Grease a 24cm round cake tin – preferably a loose-bottomed one – with butter, then sprinkle it with flour. (If you don't have a 24cm tin you can use a 22cm one and cook the cake for longer – at least an hour.)

4 Whisk the eggs in a bowl until they are frothy, then add the honey, ground almonds, baking powder and the puréed oranges. Mix thoroughly but lightly, then pour the mixture into the cake tin.

5 Bake the cake for 45–50 minutes until it's firm to touch and shrinking away from the sides of the tin. Leave it to cool in the tin before turning it out. Serve with yoghurt or crème fraiche, sweetened with a little honey if you like.

Serves 10   (F)

2 medium oranges
butter, for greasing
flour, for dusting
6 eggs
200g runny honey
350g ground almonds
1 tsp baking powder

339 calories per slice

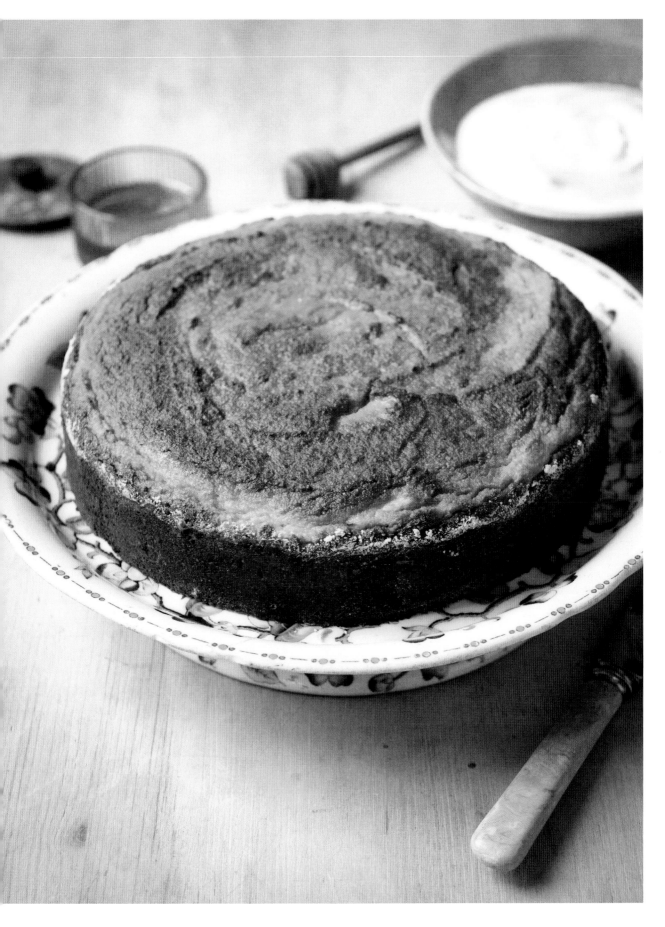

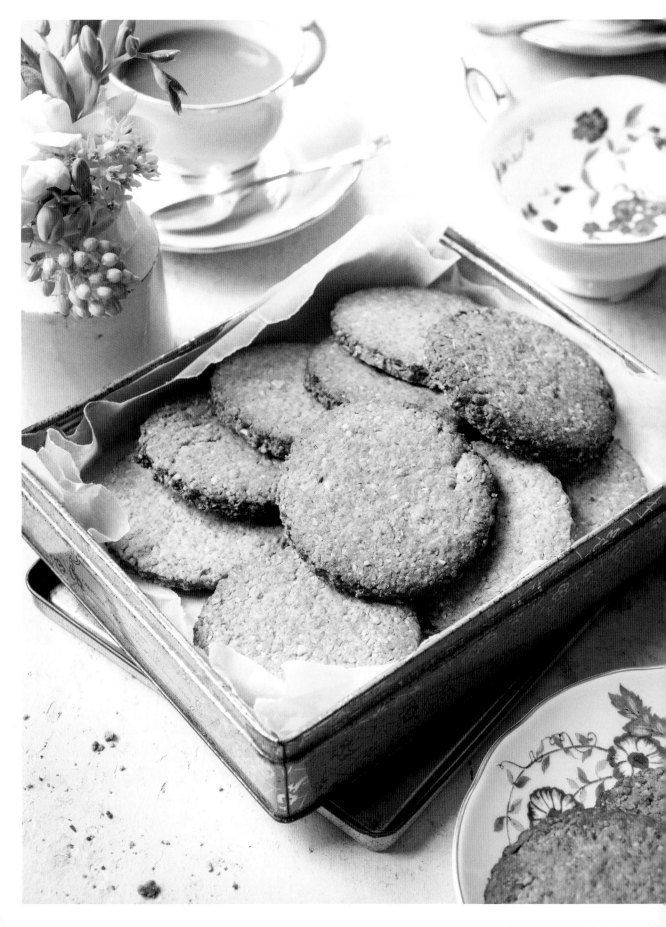

Hobby nobby biscuits

I do love a biscuit and these are made with maple syrup instead of sugar, so not as sweet as the bought kind. For a change, you could try replacing 50g of the flour with cocoa powder. The biscuits won't be quite as light but they'll still be very good.

1 Put the butter in a small saucepan and melt it over a low heat. Remove the pan from the heat and stir in the maple syrup, then set the pan aside.

2 Put the flour, oatmeal, oats, salt and baking powder in a large bowl and mix until everything is thoroughly combined. Make a well in the centre of the mixture and pour in the butter and maple syrup mixture, then gradually work in the dry ingredients until you have a coarse-textured dough. Roll the mixture into 2 balls, wrap them in cling film, then leave them to chill in the fridge for half an hour. Preheat the oven to 200°C/180°C Fan/Gas 6.

3 Roll out each ball on a lightly floured surface to a thickness of about 5mm. Using a 7cm cutter, cut out rounds of dough. If your dough is crumbly and you have problems rolling it you could press about 35–40g of the mixture into the cutter and press it down. Repeat to make each biscuit

4 Using a palette knife, carefully place the biscuits on a couple of baking trays. Bake the biscuits in the oven for 18–20 minutes until they are starting to brown round the edges. Remove the biscuits from the oven and transfer them to a cooling rack. They may feel slightly soft in the middle, but they will firm up as they cool.

Makes about 24

200g butter
175ml maple syrup
300g wholemeal flour or wholemeal spelt flour, plus extra for dusting
250g oatmeal
50g porridge oats
small pinch of salt
2 tsp baking powder

175 calories per biscuit

Apple snow

My amazing Granny Pippy used to make apple snow for me when I was a child and it still makes me feel loved! Coxes or any eating apples that soften and collapse when cooked are fine for this, but it's best to avoid cooking apples, as they need so much sweetness added.

1 Peel, core and slice the apples – you need about 500g prepared weight. Put them in a saucepan with the lemon juice and enough water to coat the bottom of the pan. Cover the pan and cook the apples over a low heat for 10–15 minutes, until they have puffed up and softened, checking them regularly to make sure they are not sticking.

2 Remove the pan from the heat and allow the apples to cool a little. Blitz them in a blender or food processor until smooth, then taste and add a little maple syrup if you think the mixture needs some extra sweetness – it shouldn't.

3 Put the egg whites in a bowl and whisk them to stiff peaks. In a separate bowl, whisk the cream until it's thick and airy, then fold both the cream and egg whites into the cooled apple mixture.

4 Spoon the mixture into serving bowls or glasses and chill them until you are ready to serve. Dust with cinnamon if you like.

Serves 4

7–8 eating apples
juice of ½ lemon
maple syrup, to taste, no
    more than 1 tbsp (optional)
2 egg whites
75ml double cream
pinch of cinnamon (optional)

157 calories per serving

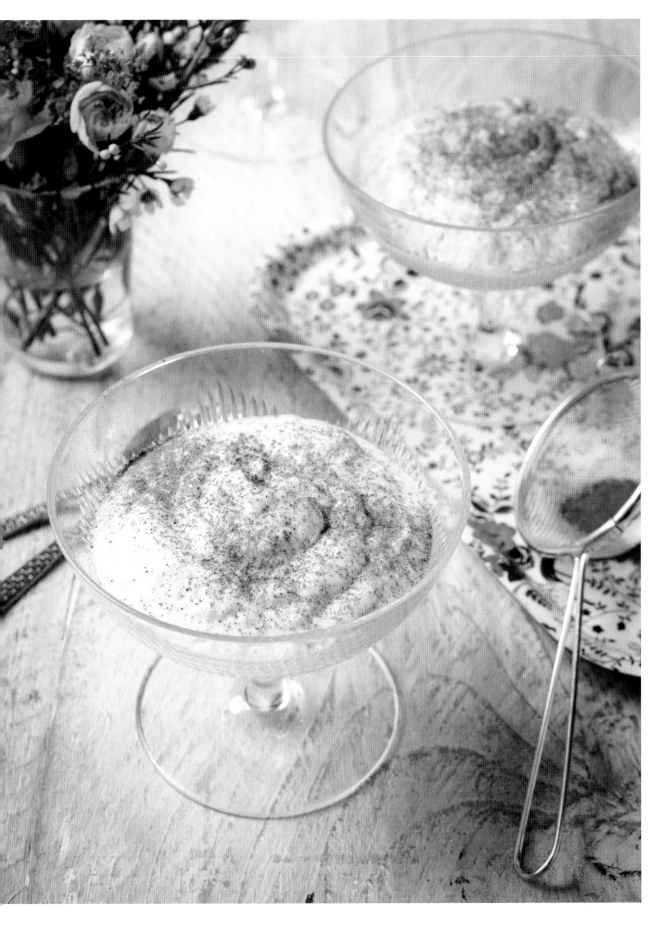

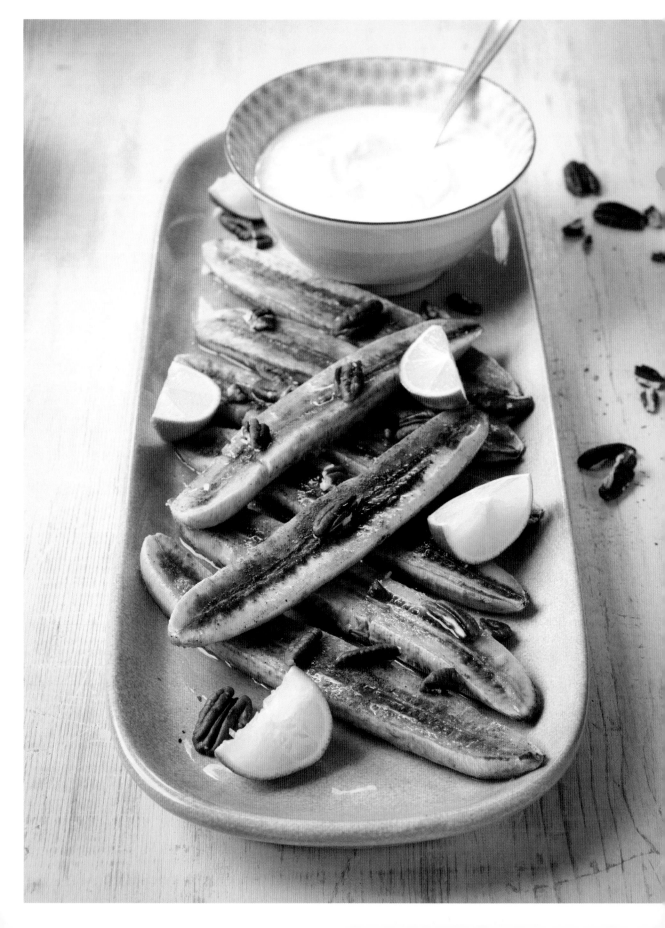

Baked bananas

Here's a super-fast pud. You can have it in the oven in no time and it tastes really comforting and luxurious.

1 Preheat the oven to 200°C/180°C Fan/Gas 6. Line a baking tray with foil and spray it very lightly with olive oil spray. Arrange the bananas on the baking tray.

2 Drizzle the bananas with maple syrup and sprinkle over the cinnamon or mixed spice. Bake the bananas in the oven for about 15 minutes until they are soft and starting to brown.

3 Transfer the bananas to a serving plate or individual bowls and spoon over any juices that have collected on the foil. Squeeze a little lime juice on each serving and top with some nuts. Serve with yoghurt, crème fraiche or frozen yoghurt.

Serves 4

olive oil spray
4 bananas, peeled and sliced
   in half lengthways
20ml maple syrup
pinch of cinnamon or mixed spice
squeeze of lime

To serve
25g pecans, chopped or crumbled
Greek yoghurt, crème fraiche or
   frozen yoghurt

148 calories per serving

Chocolate and nut spread

This is my home-made version of a very popular Italian spread. I know it's a different colour from the bought stuff, but that's because it's made with lovely, dark 100 per cent cocoa powder. I use smooth nut butter, but you could make it with the same amount of nuts instead. Be sure to use salt-free nut butter – the salty ones just don't taste right at all. The calorie count is for a serving of about one teaspoon (about 10 grams) by the way, not for the whole jar so don't be tempted to go mad!

1 Put the ingredients in a bowl and mix them until smooth, making sure the cocoa powder is completely incorporated. If you prefer, put everything in a food processor instead and blend. Decant the mixture into a clean, sterilised jar.

2 This is fine stored out of the fridge and will keep its spreadable texture. If you put it in the fridge it will firm up, so take it out for a while before using so it becomes spreadable again.

Makes 1 jar

200g smooth nut butter,
    preferably hazelnut but
    any nut butter is fine
25g cocoa powder
100ml maple syrup

50 calories per 10g serving

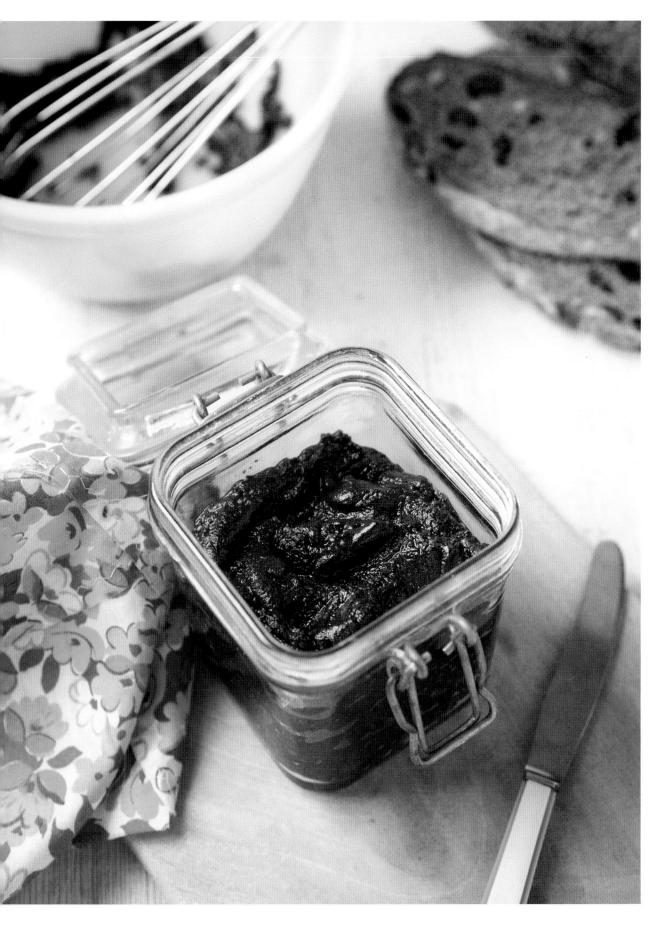

Cooking Tips

You can buy chickpeas and other pulses in cans, and ready-cooked quinoa and spelt are available in sachets, but it's far cheaper to cook your own. And it's well worth cooking up big batches of beans, chickpeas or spelt, then stashing them in the freezer for quick meals another day.

How to cook quinoa

Quinoa absorbs about two and half times its weight in liquid so 100g of raw quinoa makes about 350g cooked quinoa.

100g quinoa
250ml stock or water
salt

1 If you have time, soak the quinoa in cold water for 5 minutes. If not, put the quinoa in a sieve and run it under cold water for at least 30 seconds to remove any trace of bitterness. Drain it as thoroughly as you can, then put it in a saucepan.

2 Stir the quinoa over a medium-high heat for a couple of minutes to toast it and develop the nutty flavour, then pour over the stock or water. Season with salt. Bring it to the boil, turn the heat down to a simmer and cover the pan. Leave the quinoa to cook for 15 minutes, by which time the liquid should be absorbed.

3 Remove the pan from the heat and leave the quinoa to stand for another 5 minutes. The quinoa is now ready to use.

How to cook spelt

Spelt absorbs twice its weight in liquid, so 250g of uncooked spelt gives you about 750g of cooked spelt. You can halve this recipe if you like, but spelt freezes well so it's worth making quite a large amount. If you want to make a slightly more substantial side dish, finely chop an onion, a stick of celery and a carrot and fry them for a few minutes in the olive oil before adding the spelt.

250g uncooked spelt
1 tsp olive oil
bouquet garni (sprigs of
    parsley, thyme and bay
    leaves tied together)
1 litre chicken or vegetable stock
    or water
salt and black pepper

1 Rinse the spelt thoroughly and drain it. Heat the oil in a saucepan, then add the spelt and stir over a medium heat for 2–3 minutes. Add the herbs and the stock or water and season with salt and pepper.

2 Bring the stock to the boil, then turn the heat down to a simmer and cook the spelt for 18–20 minutes. The spelt should have softened but the grains should still have a slight bite to them. Drain and reserve the cooking liquid to use as stock for soups, if you like. The spelt can be kept in the fridge for a few days and also freezes well. To freeze, put the spelt in a freezer bag or plastic box. It defrosts almost immediately in just-boiled water.

How to cook chickpeas

Dried chickpeas make slightly more than double their weight once cooked, so 100g of dried chickpeas makes about 220g of cooked. You can increase this basic recipe as you need to and it's worth cooking a big batch, as chickpeas freeze well.

100g dried chickpeas
a couple of bay leaves (optional)
a couple of slices of onion (optional)
salt

1 Put the chickpeas in a large bowl and cover them with at least double their volume of water. Leave them to soak overnight, stirring every so often just to make sure they soak evenly. Discard any floating or discoloured chickpeas.

2 Drain the chickpeas and transfer them to a large saucepan that has a lid. Pour in enough water to come 2–3cm above the chickpeas and add the bay leaves and onion slices, if using. Bring the water to the boil and leave the chickpeas to boil hard for 10 minutes, then reduce the temperature, cover the pan with a lid and leave them to cook over a medium heat for about an hour and half. Check every so often to make sure there is enough water and top it up with boiling water if necessary. The chickpeas may take slightly longer – this depends on how old they are when you cook them, so don't worry if they aren't cooked within this time – just keep going until they are.

3 When the chickpeas are cooked, add about 1 teaspoon of salt and leave them to stand in the water for a few minutes. Drain, removing the bay leaves and onion slices. You can reserve the liquid for cooking other dishes if you like. The chickpeas will keep up to a week in the fridge. To freeze, put the chickpeas in a freezer bag or plastic box. They defrost almost immediately in just-boiled water.

4 You can cook dried beans in the same way as above, but they may not need to be boiled for as long as chickpeas.

Side dish calorie counts

Brown rice
40g (uncooked weight): 147 kcals/30g carbs

Sweet potato
200g (baked): 250 kcals/53g carbs

Quinoa
40g (uncooked weight): 131 kcals/21g carbs

Wholewheat pasta
40g (uncooked weight) wholewheat spaghetti/pasta: 144 kcals/26g carbs

Bread
1 medium slice of wholemeal bread (37g): 88 kcals/15g carbs
Small wholemeal roll (50g): 119 kcals/20g carbs
1 slice of rye bread/pumpernickle (25g) – 60 kcals/11g carbs

Nutritional Information

On the following pages you'll find a detailed nutritional breakdown for all the recipes in this book. These are estimates only and may vary depending on the ingredients used. Unless otherwise specified, the figures are per serving. Optional ingredients are not included in the analysis, but where necessary we've noted calories for extras on the recipe pages.

Kcals refers to the calories, or energy, in food. The calorie counts for all the recipes are in kcals (kilocalories). You may also see the measurement Kj (kilojoules) on packaging. This is just a different way of measuring energy and not something you need worry about.

Protein We need protein for the growth and repair of tissues in the body. Meat, poultry, fish, eggs, dairy products, nuts and pulses are all good sources of protein. New research suggests that protein can help you feel fuller for longer.

Carbs If you've had a look at the introduction you'll know that not all carbs are bad for you. Smart carbs – the unrefined, wholegrain, low GI carbs used in the recipes in this book – should be an important part of our diet, even when trying to lose weight

Sugar The figures given for sugar in the tables are for total sugar, which includes the natural sugars in foods such as fruit, vegetables, milk and yoghurt. It's the free sugars – sugar added to food – that we should be cutting back on and we've kept that type of sugar as low as possible in these recipes.

Fat The figures for fat means the total fat content, including monounsaturated and polyunsaturated fats and saturated fat. Monounsaturated fats are found in nuts and seeds, olive and rapeseed oil, and polyunsaturated fats in oily fish and vegetable oils. They are healthier types of fat but still high in calories. Experts recommend that fat should account for no more than 35 per cent of our total calorie intake each day. For women eating 2,000 calories this works out at no more than 70g per day.

Saturated fats are found in foods such as fatty cuts of meat, butter and cheese. A diet high in saturated fat has been shown to increase the risk of heart disease, which is why experts recommend that women should eat no more than 20g per day. Men can have 30g.

Fibre This is a substance found in plant foods that cannot be completely broken down by digestion. Foods such as fruit, vegetables, nuts, seeds and pulses, as well as cereals like wheat, rice, maize, corn and barley, all contain fibre. When cereals are refined some of the fibre is removed. A high-fibre diet has been shown to reduce the risk of heart disease, stroke, type 2 diabetes and certain types of cancer. A recent report suggests that adults need about 30g of fibre a day, about 50 per cent more than most people currently eat.

Salt A high salt intake is linked with high blood pressure, which is why health experts say we should have no more than 6g per day. The figure for salt given for the recipes is based on the ingredients in the recipe but does not include the salt added as seasoning to taste.

The following table shows the recommended daily amount of these various nutrients for different calorie intakes. These figures are not a target but simply guidelines.

Kcals	2,500 kcals	2,000 kcals	1,400 kcals	1,200 kcals
Protein (g)	55	45	45	45
Carbs (g)	300	270	190	160
Sugar (g)	120	90	63	54
Fat (g)	90	70	49	42
Saturated fat (g)	30	20	14	12
Fibre (g)	30	30	30	30
Salt (g)	6	6	6	6

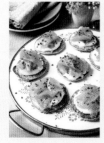

Buckwheat blinis
Page 18
(per blini)
Kcals 60
Protein (g) 2.5
Carbs (g) 8
Sugar (g) 1
Fat (g) 2
Saturated fat (g) 0.6
Fibre (g) 0.5
Salt (g) 0.2

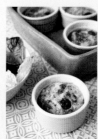

Pastryless quiches
Page 21
(per quiche)
Kcals 170
Protein (g) 9.5
Carbs (g) 0.7
Sugar (g) 0.6
Fat (g) 14
Saturated fat (g) 7
Fibre (g) 0.1
Salt (g) 0.4

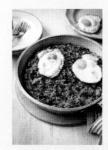

Bubble & squeak
Page 22
Kcals 119
Protein (g) 3
Carbs (g) 11
Sugar (g) 10
Fat (g) 6
Saturated fat (g) 2
Fibre (g) 6.5
Salt (g) 0.2

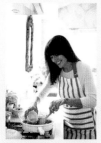

Veggie shakshuka
Page 25
Kcals 215
Protein (g) 13
Carbs (g) 13
Sugar (g) 13
Fat (g) 11
Saturated fat (g) 4
Fibre (g) 4
Salt (g) 0.6

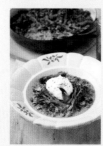

Beans & eggs
Page 26
Kcals 522
Protein (g) 24
Carbs (g) 30
Sugar (g) 9.5
Fat (g) 30
Saturated fat (g) 18
Fibre (g) 15
Salt (g) 1

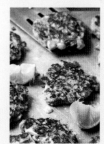

Sweetcorn fritters
Page 29
(per fritter)
Kcals 37
Protein (g) 1.5
Carbs (g) 4
Sugar (g) 0.8
Fat (g) 1.5
Saturated fat (g) 0.3
Fibre (g) 0.7
Salt (g) 0.3

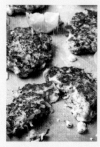

Courgette & feta fritters
Page 29
(per fritter)
Kcals 53
Protein (g) 3.3
Carbs (g) 3
Sugar (g) 0.5
Fat (g) 3
Saturated fat (g) 1.5
Fibre (g) 0.7
Salt (g) 0.2

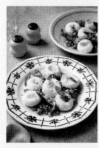

Ricotta dumplings
Page 30
(with tomato sauce/
*with butter sauce)
Kcals 436/*412
Protein (g) 17/*17
Carbs (g) 51/*48
Sugar (g) 5.5/*2
Fat (g) 17/*17
Sat fat (g) 7.6/*10
Fibre (g) 3/*2
Salt (g) 0.3/*0.4

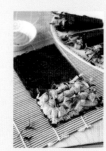

Salmon hand rolls
Page 33
Kcals 124
Protein (g) 7
Carbs (g) 10
Sugar (g) 2
Fat (g) 6
Saturated fat (g) 1
Fibre (g) 2
Salt (g) 0.4

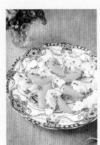

Citrus chilli fish
Page 34
Kcals 282
Protein (g) 31
Carbs (g) 6
Sugar (g) 6
Fat (g) 15
Saturated fat (g) 3
Fibre (g) 1
Salt (g) 0.3

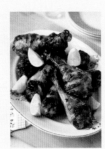

Buttermilk chicken
Page 37
Kcals 262
Protein (g) 37
Carbs (g) 0.5
Sugar (g) 0.5
Fat (g) 14
Saturated fat (g) 4
Fibre (g) 0
Salt (g) 0.4

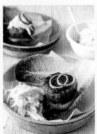

Pork sliders & quick apple coleslaw
Page 38
Kcals 337
Protein (g) 30
Carbs (g) 16
Sugar (g) 7
Fat (g) 16
Saturated fat (g) 6
Fibre (g) 3.5
Salt (g) 0.5

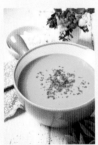

Carrot, celeriac & coriander soup
Page 42
(feta adds 30 kcals per serving)
Kcals 125
Protein (g) 11
Carbs (g) 9
Sugar (g) 7.5
Fat (g) 4
Saturated fat (g) 1.8
Fibre (g) 6
Salt (g) 0.8

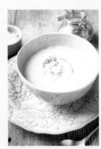

Cauliflower cheese soup
Page 45
Kcals 219
Protein (g) 18
Carbs (g) 12.5
Sugar (g) 9
Fat (g) 10
Saturated fat (g) 6
Fibre (g) 4.5
Salt (g) 0.9

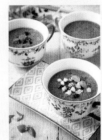

Gazpacho
Page 46
(without garnishes)
Kcals 213
Protein (g) 6
Carbs (g) 15
Sugar (g) 15
Fat (g) 13
Saturated fat (g) 2
Fibre (g) 7
Salt (g) 0.4

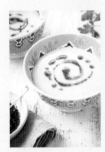

White bean & parsley soup
Page 49
Kcals 417
Protein (g) 35
Carbs (g) 36
Sugar (g) 4
Fat (g) 11
Saturated fat (g) 2
Fibre (g) 16
Salt (g) 3.5

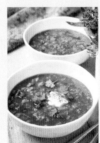

Red lentil, squash & tomato soup
Page 50
Kcals 259
Protein (g) 20
Carbs (g) 33
Sugar (g) 10.5
Fat (g) 4
Saturated fat (g) 0.8
Fibre (g) 5
Salt (g) 0.6

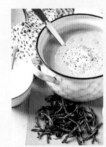

Sweetcorn chowder
Page 53
Kcals 276
Protein (g) 21
Carbs (g) 17
Sugar (g) 6
Fat (g) 12
Saturated fat (g) 5
Fibre (g) 4.5
Salt (g) 1.5

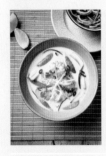

Thai prawn & coconut soup
Page 54
(with noodles/*with spiralised courgettes)
Kcals 331/*278
Protein (g) 17/*19
Carbs (g) 23/*8
Sugar (g) 3/*4
Fat (g) 18/*18
Sat fat (g) 15/*15
Fibre (g) 3/*2.5
Salt (g) 2/*1.7

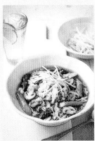

Asian crab & asparagus soup
Page 57
Kcals 171
Protein (g) 19
Carbs (g) 13
Sugar (g) 3.5
Fat (g) 4.5
Saturated fat (g) 1
Fibre (g) 2.5
Salt (g) 1.2

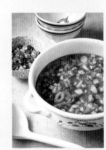

Summer chicken broth
Page 58
Kcals 255
Protein (g) 33
Carbs (g) 9
Sugar (g) 7
Fat (g) 8.5
Saturated fat (g) 2.5
Fibre (g) 5.5
Salt (g) 0.7

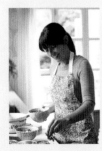

Tex-Mex chicken soup
Page 61
Kcals 394
Protein (g) 30
Carbs (g) 30
Sugar (g) 10.5
Fat (g) 15
Saturated fat (g) 3.5
Fibre (g) 11
Salt (g) 0.6

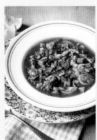

Lamb & barley soup
Page 62
Kcals 357
Protein (g) 34
Carbs (g) 20
Sugar (g) 11
Fat (g) 13
Saturated fat (g) 4.5
Fibre (g) 13
Salt (g) 0.8

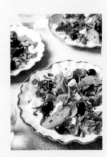

Couscous, orange & goat's cheese salad
Page 66
Kcals 333
Protein (g) 12
Carbs (g) 34
Sugar (g) 9
Fat (g) 15.5
Saturated fat (g) 6
Fibre (g) 5.5
Salt (g) 0.2

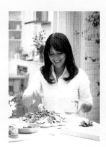

Californian salad
Page 69
Kcals 175
Protein (g) 4
Carbs (g) 16
Sugar (g) 15
Fat (g) 9
Saturated fat (g) 0.7
Fibre (g) 6.5
Salt (g) 1

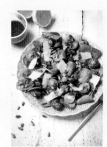

Mushroom, spinach & tomato salad
Page 70
Kcals 161
Protein (g) 7
Carbs (g) 3
Sugar (g) 3
Fat (g) 12.5
Saturated fat (g) 2.5
Fibre (g) 3
Salt (g) 0.3

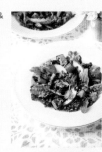

Pumpkin & lentil salad
Page 73
Kcals 269
Protein (g) 13
Carbs (g) 25
Sugar (g) 13
Fat (g) 11.5
Saturated fat (g) 2.5
Fibre (g) 0.8
Salt (g) 0.9

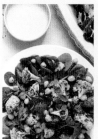

Mediterranean roasted vegetable salad
Page 74
Kcals 190
Protein (g) 11
Carbs (g) 23
Sugar (g) 11
Fat (g) 4
Saturated fat (g) 0.7
Fibre (g) 10
Salt (g) 0.2

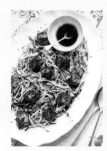

Marinated salmon with Asian coleslaw
Page 75
Kcals 320
Protein (g) 32
Carbs (g) 6.5
Sugar (g) 5
Fat (g) 17.5
Saturated fat (g) 3.5
Fibre (g) 4
Salt (g) 2.2

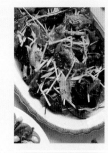

Smoked fish & beetroot salad
Page 75
Kcals 308
Protein (g) 17
Carbs (g) 15
Sugar (g) 14
Fat (g) 19
Saturated fat (g) 3.5
Fibre (g) 6
Salt (g) 1.7

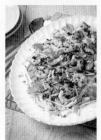

Thai prawn salad
Page 78
Kcals 115
Protein (g) 10
Carbs (g) 8
Sugar (g) 8
Fat (g) 4
Saturated fat (g) 0.6
Fibre (g) 3
Salt (g) 1.8

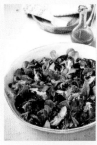

Harissa chicken & freekeh salad
Page 81
Kcals 283
Protein (g) 27
Carbs (g) 24
Sugar (g) 6
Fat (g) 7.5
Saturated fat (g) 1.5
Fibre (g) 6
Salt (g) 0.4

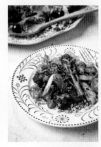

Chicken, broccoli & spelt salad
Page 82
Kcals 286
Protein (g) 30
Carbs (g) 21
Sugar (g) 5
Fat (g) 7.5
Saturated fat (g) 1.5
Fibre (g) 6.5
Salt (g) 1.4

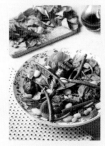

Garlic sausage & bean salad
Page 85
Kcals 276
Protein (g) 15
Carbs (g) 16
Sugar (g) 3.5
Fat (g) 14.5
Saturated fat (g) 4
Fibre (g) 10
Salt (g) 1

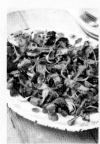

Beef salad with sundried tomatoes
Page 86
Kcals 322
Protein (g) 39
Carbs (g) 3
Sugar (g) 2.5
Fat (g) 16.5
Saturated fat (g) 4.5
Fibre (g) 3
Salt (g) 0.5

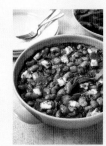

Greek giant beans
Page 90
(per 200g serving)
Kcals 144
Protein (g) 8
Carbs (g) 20
Sugar (g) 5
Fat (g) 2
Saturated fat (g) 1
Fibre (g) 8
Salt (g) trace

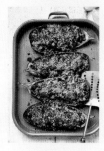

Stuffed aubergines
Page 93
Kcals 261
Protein (g) 11
Carbs (g) 21
Sugar (g) 8
Fat (g) 13
Saturated fat (g) 2.5
Fibre (g) 10
Salt (g) 0.3

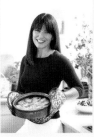

Davina's special lasagne
Page 94
(serves 4/*serves 6)
Kcals 538/*358
Protein (g) 25/*16
Carbs (g) 60/*40
Sugar (g) 15/*10
Fat (g) 20/*13
Sat fat (g) 10/*6.5
Fibre (g) 9/*6
Salt (g) 1.5/*0.9

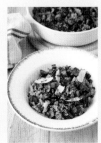

Veggie quinoa risotto
Page 97
Kcals 278
Protein (g) 12
Carbs (g) 33
Sugar (g) 6
Fat (g) 10
Saturated fat (g) 3
Fibre (g) 5
Salt (g) 0.3

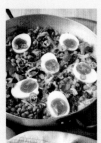

Spinach & egg curry
Page 98
Kcals 371
Protein (g) 16
Carbs (g) 12
Sugar (g) 5.5
Fat (g) 27
Saturated fat (g) 18
Fibre (g) 5
Salt (g) 0.4

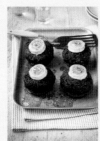

Quinoa & sweet potato burgers
Page 101
Kcals 330
Protein (g) 13
Carbs (g) 33
Sugar (g) 8
Fat (g) 12
Saturated fat (g) 5
Fibre (g) 5
Salt (g) 0.6

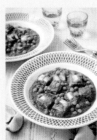

Paneer & pea curry
Page 102
Kcals 439
Protein (g) 22
Carbs (g) 33
Sugar (g) 30
Fat (g) 24
Saturated fat (g) 13.5
Fibre (g) 3
Salt (g) 0.6

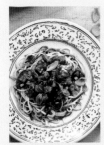

Fresh tomato sauce with pasta
Page 104
(*with courgetti)
Kcals 260/*105
Protein (g) 8/*4
Carbs (g) 36/*6
Sugar (g) 5.5/*5.5
Fat (g) 7.5/*7
Saturated fat (g) 1.5/*1.5
Fibre (g) 7/*3
Salt (g) 0.1/*0.1

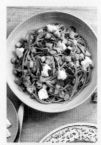

Ricotta & herb sauce with pasta
Page 104
Kcals 317
Protein (g) 13
Carbs (g) 36
Sugar (g) 4
Fat (g) 11.5
Saturated fat (g) 4
Fibre (g) 9
Salt (g) 0.4

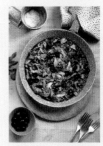

Tuna pasta sauce with pasta
Page 105
(*with courgetti)
Kcals 260/*105
Protein (g) 14/*10
Carbs (g) 36/*5
Sugar (g) 4/*4.5
Fat (g) 5/*4.5
Sat fat (g) 0.8/*0.8
Fibre (g) 7/*2.5
Salt (g) 0.4/*0.4

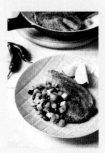

Blackened fish with bean & avocado salsa
Page 108
Kcals 427
Protein (g) 37
Carbs (g) 27
Sugar (g) 7
Fat (g) 16.5
Saturated fat (g) 3.5
Fibre (g) 11
Salt (g) 1.8

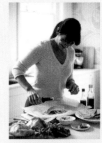

Roasted fish with braised cabbage & bacon
Page 111
Kcals 400
Protein (g) 41
Carbs (g) 14
Sugar (g) 4
Fat (g) 18
Saturated fat (g) 9
Fibre (g) 7.5
Salt (g) 1.5

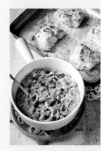

Chinese fish parcels
Page 112
Kcals 175
Protein (g) 29
Carbs (g) 7
Sugar (g) 6.5
Fat (g) 2
Saturated fat (g) 0.5
Fibre (g) 4
Salt (g) 2.6

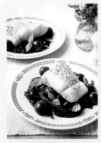

Fish Provençal
Page 115
Kcals 217
Protein (g) 28
Carbs (g) 7
Sugar (g) 6.5
Fat (g) 8
Saturated fat (g) 1.5
Fibre (g) 3
Salt (g) 0.6

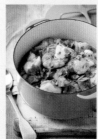

Seafood tagine
Page 116
Kcals 198
Protein (g) 36
Carbs (g) 3
Sugar (g) 2.5
Fat (g) 4
Saturated fat (g) 0.7
Fibre (g) 3
Salt (g) 2

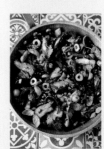

Spanish chicken
Page 120
Kcals 220
Protein (g) 28
Carbs (g) 7
Sugar (g) 5
Fat (g) 9
Saturated fat (g) 2
Fibre (g) 2
Salt (g) 1.7

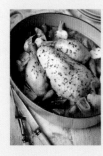

Poached chicken with lemon sauce
Page 123
Kcals 386
Protein (g) 62
Carbs (g) 11
Sugar (g) 9
Fat (g) 9
Saturated fat (g) 4
Fibre (g) 8
Salt (g) 0.5

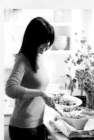

Chicken crumble
Page 124
Kcals 471
Protein (g) 45
Carbs (g) 32
Sugar (g) 11
Fat (g) 16
Saturated fat (g) 6.5
Fibre (g) 9
Salt (g) 0.8

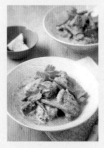

Chicken curry
Page 127
Kcals 337
Protein (g) 41
Carbs (g) 9
Sugar (g) 5
Fat (g) 14.5
Saturated fat (g) 2.5
Fibre (g) 3.5
Salt (g) 0.9

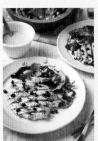

Grilled chicken with tahini sauce
Page 128
Kcals 320
Protein (g) 42
Carbs (g) 0.5
Sugar (g) 0.5
Fat (g) 16.5
Saturated fat (g) 2.5
Fibre (g) 3
Salt (g) 0.2

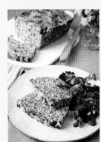

Chicken meatloaf
Page 131
(serves 4/*serves 6)
Kcals 393/*262
Protein (g) 55/*37
Carbs (g) 19/*12.5
Sugar (g) 5/*3.5
Fat (g) 10/*7
Saturated fat (g) 4/*2.5
Fibre (g) 3.3/*2.2
Salt (g) 0.7/*0.5

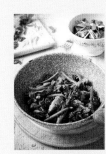

Vietnamese chicken stir-fry
Page 132
Kcals 223
Protein (g) 40
Carbs (g) 3
Sugar (g) 2
Fat (g) 5
Saturated fat (g) 0.8
Fibre (g) 3.5
Salt (g) 1.2

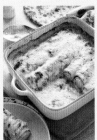

Leek & ham gratin
Page 135
Kcals 303
Protein (g) 21
Carbs (g) 15
Sugar (g) 10
Fat (g) 16
Saturated fat (g) 9
Fibre (g) 7
Salt (g) 1.6

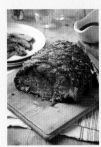

Slow-roast pork with braised fennel
Page 136
(*without crackling)
Kcals 480/*411
Protein (g) 67/*66
Carbs (g) 2/*2
Sugar (g) 2/*2
Fat (g) 22/*15
Saturated fat (g) 7/*4.5
Fibre (g) 2/*2
Salt (g) 0.5/*0.5

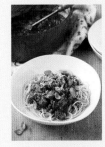

Pork ragu
Page 139
(Serves 6/*serves 8)
Kcals 472/*400
Protein (g) 45/*36
Carbs (g) 42/*39
Sugar (g) 10/*8
Fat (g) 12/*9
Saturated fat (g) 3/*2.5
Fibre (g) 9/*8
Salt (g) 0.3/*0.25

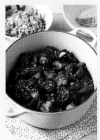

Lamb & aubergine casserole
Page 140
Kcals 334
Protein (g) 33
Carbs (g) 13
Sugar (g) 11
Fat (g) 16
Saturated fat (g) 6
Fibre (g) 6
Salt (g) 0.3

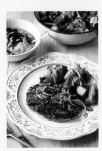

Greek lamb
Page 143
Kcals 387
Protein (g) 35
Carbs (g) 8
Sugar (g) 7.5
Fat (g) 23
Saturated fat (g) 9.5
Fibre (g) 2.5
Salt (g) 0.4

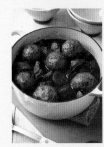

Beef casserole with squash and chestnut dumplings
Page 144
(Serves 4/*serves 6
Kcals 602/*401
Protein (g) 50/*33
Carbs (g) 32/*21
Sugar (g) 11/*7.5
Fat (g) 24/*16
Saturated fat (g) 10/*7
Fibre (g) 7/*4.5
Salt (g) 0.9/*0.6

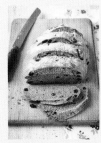

Walnut & raisin bread
Page 148
(per slice – 16 slices)
Kcals 161
Protein (g) 4.5
Carbs (g) 25
Sugar (g) 4
Fat (g) 4
Saturated fat (g) 0.4
Fibre (g) 4
Salt (g) 0.4

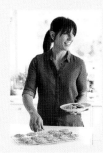

Spelt & rye crackers
Page 151
(per cracker with seeds/
*per cracker with cheese)
Kcals 61/*55
Protein (g) 2/*1.7
Carbs (g) 9/*9
Sugar (g) 0.1/*0.1
Fat (g) 1.5/*1
Sat fat (g) 0.3/*0.4
Fibre (g) 1/*0.9
Salt (g) 0.1/*0.1

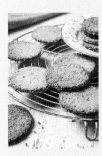

Oatcakes
Page 152
(per oatcake)
Kcals 96
Protein (g) 2
Carbs (g) 10
Sugar (g) 0.1
Fat (g) 5
Saturated fat (g) 3
Fibre (g) 1.5
Salt (g) 0.2

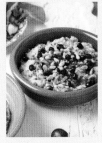

Aubergine dip
Page 155
(per 30g serving)
Kcals 20
Protein (g) 0.5
Carbs (g) 1
Sugar (g) 0.7
Fat (g) 1.5
Saturated fat (g) 0
Fibre (g) 1
Salt (g) 0

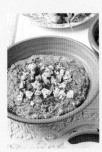

Roast red pepper & feta dip
Page 155
(per 30g serving)
Kcals 34
Protein (g) 1.5
Carbs (g) 1
Sugar (g) 1
Fat (g) 2.5
Saturated fat (g) 1.5
Fibre (g) 0.5
Salt (g) 0.2

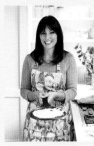

Chickpea flatbreads
Page 156
(per large flatbread/
*per small flatbread)
Kcals 141/*94
Protein (g) 9/*6
Carbs (g) 20/*14
Sugar (g) 0.8/*0.5
Fat (g) 2/*1.5
Sat fat (g) 0.2/*0.2
Fibre (g) 4/*2.5
Salt (g) 0.6/*0.4

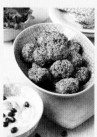

Broad bean falafel
Page 159
Kcals 292
Protein (g) 13
Carbs (g) 20
Sugar (g) 8
Fat (g) 16
Saturated fat (g) 5
Fibre (g) 10.5
Salt (g) 0.4

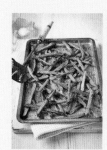

Sweet potato fries
Page 160
Kcals 195
Protein (g) 1.5
Carbs (g) 32
Sugar (g) 7
Fat (g) 6
Saturated fat (g) 1
Fibre (g) 4
Salt (g) 0.1

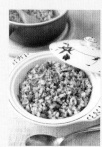

Braised barley
Page 163
Kcals 347
Protein (g) 18
Carbs (g) 57
Sugar (g) 6
Fat (g) 4.5
Saturated fat (g) 1
Fibre (g) 3
Salt (g) 0.7

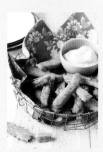

Chickpea flour chips
Page 164
Kcals 240
Protein (g) 8
Carbs (g) 20
Sugar (g) 1
Fat (g) 13
Saturated fat (g) 2
Fibre (g) 4
Salt (g) 0

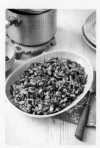

Brown rice pilaf
Page 167
Kcals 186
Protein (g) 8
Carbs (g) 27
Sugar (g) 3
Fat (g) 3.5
Saturated fat (g) 0.5
Fibre (g) 6
Salt (g) 0.1

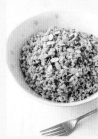

Vegetable couscous
Page 168
Kcals 76
Protein (g) 4
Carbs (g) 6
Sugar (g) 4
Fat (g) 3
Saturated fat (g) 0.5
Fibre (g) 3
Salt (g) 0

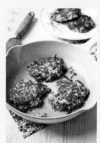

Parsnip rösti
Page 171
Kcals 107
Protein (g) 3
Carbs (g) 11
Sugar (g) 7
Fat (g) 5
Saturated fat (g) 1
Fibre (g) 3
Salt (g) 0.1

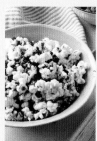

Popcorn
Page 172
(*sweet popcorn)
Kcals 75/*92
Protein (g) 2/*2
Carbs (g) 12/*17
Sugar (g) 0/*4
Fat (g) 2/*2
Sat fat (g) 0.1/*0.1
Fibre (g) 0.5/*0.5
Salt (g) 0/*0

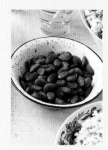

Smoky almonds
Page 173
(per 20g serving)
Kcals 142
Protein (g) 5
Carbs (g) 1
Sugar (g) 0.8
Fat (g) 12
Saturated fat (g) 1
Fibre (g) 10
Salt (g) 0.3

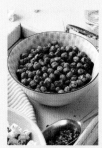

Roasted chickpeas
Page 173
(per 50g serving)
Kcals 71
Protein (g) 4
Carbs (g) 6
Sugar (g) 0
Fat (g) 3
Saturated fat (g) 4
Fibre (g) 4
Salt (g) 0

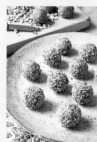

Apricot & pistachio power balls
Page 176
Kcals 106
Protein (g) 3.5
Carbs (g) 6
Sugar (g) 5
Fat (g) 7.5
Saturated fat (g) 3
Fibre (g) 2
Salt (g) 0.1

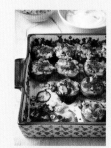

Baked plums
Page 180
Kcals 414
Protein (g) 8
Carbs (g) 15
Sugar (g) 15
Fat (g) 35
Saturated fat (g) 15
Fibre (g) 2
Salt (g) 0.2

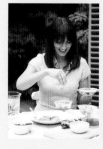

Poached peaches with pistachios
Page 183
Kcals 200
Protein (g) 3
Carbs (g) 29
Sugar (g) 29
Fat (g) 7
Saturated fat (g) 1
Fibre (g) 3
Salt (g) 0

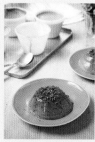

Chocolate panna cotta
Page 184
Kcals 418
Protein (g) 5
Carbs (g) 27
Sugar (g) 27
Fat (g) 32
Saturated fat (g) 20
Fibre (g) 0
Salt (g) 0.1

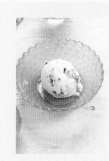

Frozen yoghurt
Page 186
Kcals 214
Protein (g) 7
Carbs (g) 18
Sugar (g) 16
Fat (g) 13
Saturated fat (g) 8.5
Fibre (g) 0
Salt (g) 0.2

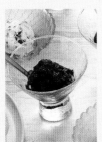

Watermelon & cherry slush
Page 186
Kcals 110
Protein (g) 1
Carbs (g) 26
Sugar (g) 26
Fat (g) 0
Saturated fat (g) 0
Fibre (g) 0.8
Salt (g) 0

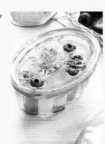

Coconut water jelly
Page 187
Kcals 47
Protein (g) 1
Carbs (g) 9
Sugar (g) 9
Fat (g) 0.5
Saturated fat (g) 0.3
Fibre (g) 0.6
Salt (g) 0.3

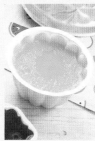

Orange & lime juice jelly
Page 187
Kcals 47
Protein (g) 1.5
Carbs (g) 10
Sugar (g) 10
Fat (g) 0
Saturated fat (g) 0
Fibre (g) 0
Salt (g) 0

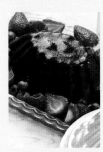

Fruits of the forest jelly
Page 187
Kcals 71
Protein (g) 2
Carbs (g) 13
Sugar (g) 13
Fat (g) 0
Saturated fat (g) 0
Fibre (g) 5
Salt (g) 0

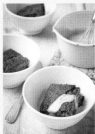

Sticky toffee pudding
Page 190
(with sauce/*without sauce)
Kcals 345/*218
Protein (g) 6/*5
Carbs (g) 41/*32
Sugar (g) 25/*17
Fat (g) 17/*7
Sat fat (g) 10/*4
Fibre (g) 3/*3
Salt (g) 0.5/*0.4

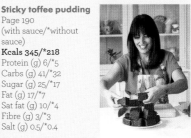

Chocolate & banana tray bake
Page 193
(per slice –16 slices)
Kcals 212
Protein (g) 5
Carbs (g) 21
Sugar (g) 10
Fat (g) 12
Saturated fat (g) 7
Fibre (g) 1.5
Salt (g) 0.4

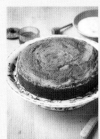

Orange & almond cake
Page 194
(per slice – 10 slices)
Kcals 339
Protein (g) 14
Carbs (g) 19
Sugar (g) 18
Fat (g) 23
Saturated fat (g) 2.5
Fibre (g) 0.5
Salt (g) 0.3

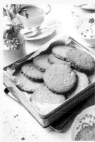

Hobby nobby biscuits
Page 197
(per biscuit)
Kcals 175
Protein (g) 3
Carbs (g) 21
Sugar (g) 4.5
Fat (g) 8
Saturated fat (g) 4.5
Fibre (g) 2.5
Salt (g) 0.4

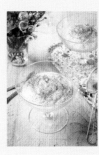

Apple snow
Page 198
Kcals 157
Protein (g) 3
Carbs (g) 12
Sugar (g) 12
Fat (g) 11
Saturated fat (g) 6.5
Fibre (g) 1
Salt (g) 0.1

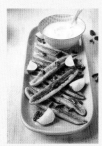

Baked bananas
Page 201
Kcals 148
Protein (g) 2
Carbs (g) 24
Sugar (g) 21
Fat (g) 5
Saturated fat (g) 0.5
Fibre (g) 2
Salt (g) 0

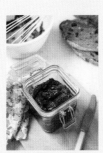

Chocolate & nut spread
Page 202
(per 10g serving)
Kcals 50
Protein (g) 2
Carbs (g) 3
Sugar (g) 2
Fat (g) 3.5
Saturated fat (g) 1
Fibre (g) 0.5
Salt (g) 0.1

My 5 Week Plan

Thinking ahead is one of the key factors in making sure you eat a healthy and balanced diet. If you're tired and frazzled at the end of a busy day it's good to have planned what you are going to cook – and it helps you not to reach for the stodge. And this plan helps you to make sure you're eating plenty of those wonderful smart carbs and including lots of fibre-rich foods to keep your body healthy.

The menus below are simply suggestions. If you want to substitute some of the meals with your own favourite dishes or recipes from 5 *Weeks to Sugar-Free*, that's fine but bear in mind the guidelines covered in the introduction: base meals around lean protein and plenty of veg, choose smart carbs and good fats. The plan is designed to help you lose weight in a safe and healthy way. At the same time, it will help you cut right back on added sugar and empty calories and gradually reduce the amount of carbs you eat – making sure those are all lovely smart carbs.

While you're following the plan it's important to drink plenty of water. First, it reduces the urge to snack or overeat. And second, the diet is designed to boost your fibre intake and without enough water fibre can't do its job (which is to keep your digestive system healthy). Other drinks like tea and coffee are allowed, but it's good to avoid sweet drinks, even the calorie-free ones, because the aim is to retrain your taste buds to enjoy the natural flavours of food and wean yourself off things that are overly sweet. Best to stop drinking alcohol for these five weeks too.

If you want to substitute your own meals, check the calories and carbs they contain, but a few calories or grams of carbs more or less each day isn't going to ruin your diet. Most of the recipes in 5 *Weeks to Sugar-Free* will work well here. Also, you can have as many green and non-starchy vegetables as you like, so eat plenty of those. You'll fill yourself up and do yourself good as well. Most of these meals are fine for the non-dieters in the family, but you'll probably want to add extra side dishes for them – and some more of the yummy smart carb puds!

Having some soups and other dishes in the freezer makes it less likely you'll get caught out and resort to the packaged stuff. Make double quantities of recipes, then freeze them for extra-busy days. You might also like to cook up big batches of standby items like spelt and chickpeas (see pages 204–205) and keep those in the freezer, ready to put together a speedy meal.

Week 1   Aim for 1,400 kcals a day. That's about 300 kcals for breakfast, 350 for lunch and 550 for your evening meal, plus a snack (about 100 calories) mid-morning and the same in the afternoon. In the weekend menus, we've allowed for a slightly bigger breakfast so dropped the snacks. If you want to count carbs as well as calories aim for about 190g of carbs a day.

Week 2   Aim for 1,300 kcals a day That's about 300 kcals for breakfast, 300 for lunch and 500 for your evening meal, plus a snack (about 100 calories) mid-morning and the same in the afternoon. If you want to count carbs as well, aim for about 175g of carbs a day.

Weeks 3, 4, 5   Aim for 1,200 kcals a day. That's about 250 kcals for breakfast, 300 for lunch and 450 for your evening meal, plus snacks. If you want to count carbs as well aim for about 160g of carbs a day.

Week 1

	Breakfast	Snack	Lunch	Snack	Evening meal
Monday	Proper porridge* + handful of blueberries	Apricot and pistachio power ball	Chicken, broccoli and spelt salad; nectarine	15g smoky almonds	Blackened fish with bean and avocado salsa + steamed green veg
Tuesday	1 slice of wholemeal toast with 2 tsp of peanut butter; 1 banana	Apple	Smoked fish and beetroot salad; 1 orange	1 rye and spelt cracker + 30g red pepper and feta dip	Poached chicken with lemon sauce + 1 x 175g baked sweet potato + French beans
Wednesday	3 tbsp sugar-free muesli + 200ml milk + handful of blueberries	100g pomegranate seeds	Tex-Mex chicken soup + 1 slice of wholegrain bread	1 oatcake + 1 tsp peanut butter	Fresh tomato sauce and pasta + 100g cooked peeled prawns
Thursday	1 boiled egg + 1 slice wholemeal toast	Banana	Marinated salmon with Asian coleslaw; apple	20g savoury popcorn	Quinoa risotto + green salad
Friday	2 slices of wholemeal toast with 10g butter + 2 slices of ham and tomato	100g fresh mango	Couscous, orange and goat's cheese salad; 100g slice of watermelon	100g roasted chickpeas	Chicken meatloaf + steamed green veg + 1 corn on the cob with 1 tsp of butter
Saturday	½ grapefruit + veggie shakshuka with 1 poached egg	-	Mediterranean roasted vegetable salad; slice of fresh pineapple	-	Slow-roast pork with braised fennel + 175g sweet potato mashed with 1 tsp butter; Apple snow
Sunday	½ grapefruit + scrambled eggs (2 medium eggs and 1 tsp butter) + 1 slice of wholemeal toast	-	Thai prawn and coconut soup + 1 wholemeal roll; slice of fresh melon	-	Beef casserole with squash and chestnut dumplings + steamed green veg; Watermelon and cherry slush

*Recipe in 5 Weeks to Sugar-Free or follow your own.

Week 2

	Breakfast	Snack	Lunch	Snack	Evening meal
Monday	Bircher muesli + 150ml milk; 1 boiled egg	Apple	Red lentil, squash and tomato soup; 1 orange	1 spelt and rye cracker + 1 tbsp hummus	Roasted fish with braised cabbage and bacon + steamed broccoli
Tuesday	150ml Greek yoghurt + 1 chopped banana	3 Brazil nuts	Harissa chicken and freekeh salad; kiwi fruit	50g olives	Chicken crumble + steamed green veg
Wednesday	3 tbsp sugar-free muesli + 200ml milk + handful of blueberries	100g pomegranate seeds	Garlic sausage and bean salad; satsuma	20g savoury popcorn	Tuna sauce and pasta; large salad + 2 tsp dressing
Thursday	2 slices of wholemeal toast + 10g butter + 2 thin slices of Edam cheese + sliced tomato	15g smoky almonds	Citrus chilli fish; fresh fruit salad	Apricot and pistachio power ball	Grilled chicken with tahini sauce + braised barley + green veg
Friday	Smoothie with 100g mango + 200ml milk + 5 tbsp Greek yoghurt	Apple	Sweetcorn chowder; 2 plums	100g roasted chickpeas	Chinese fish parcels + 50g (raw weight) brown rice
Saturday	1 slice of wholemeal toast + 2 rashers of grilled lean back bacon + mushrooms + grilled tomato	-	Beans and eggs	-	Paneer and pea curry + 30g (raw weight) brown basmati rice; Baked bananas
Sunday	Bubble and squeak + 1 poached egg	-	Californian salad	-	Lamb and aubergine casserole + vegetable couscous; Frozen yoghurt

Week 3

	Breakfast	Snack	Lunch	Snack	Evening meal
Monday	Proper porridge*	1 oatcake + 1 tbsp aubergine dip	Mediterranean roasted vegetable salad + 1 wholemeal pitta; 1 plum	Savoury popcorn	Roasted fish with braised cabbage and bacon + steamed green veg
Tuesday	125ml Greek yoghurt + 1 chopped banana	Apple	Cauliflower cheese soup + 1 slice of wholemeal bread	1 rye and spelt cracker + 1 tbsp roasted red pepper and feta dip	1 lean pork chop (grilled) + bubble and squeak + grilled tomatoes
Wednesday	2 tbsp sugar-free muesli + 200ml milk + handful of blueberries	Apricot and pistachio power ball	Pastryless quiche + Californian salad	50g roasted chickpeas	Davina's special lasagne + green salad
Thursday	1 slice of wholemeal toast + 1 poached egg + 1 slice of ham	100g fresh mango	Red lentil, squash and tomato soup; 125g plain yoghurt + seeds from 2 passion fruit	1 spelt and rye cracker + 1 tbsp aubergine dip	Buttermilk chicken + sweet potato fries + steamed green veg
Friday	Smoothie made from frozen summer fruit + 200ml milk + 5 tbsp Greek yoghurt	Banana	Asian crab and asparagus soup + spelt and rye cracker + 20g Edam cheese	50g olives	Spinach and egg curry + 30g (raw weight) brown basmati rice
Saturday	Proper porridge*	-	Broad bean falafel	-	150g rump steak + brown rice pilaf; Baked bananas
Sunday	3 courgette and feta fritters + grilled tomatoes	-	Carrot, celeriac and coriander soup + 25g croutons	-	Pork ragu + pasta; slice of fresh pineapple

*Recipe in 5 Weeks to Sugar-Free or follow your own.

Week 4

	Breakfast	Snack	Lunch	Snack	Evening meal
Monday	150ml Greek yoghurt + 1 chopped banana	15g almonds	Summer chicken broth; pear	Apple	Stuffed aubergines + 1 wholemeal pitta
Tuesday	100ml Greek yoghurt + 100ml milk + 30g sugar-free muesli	100g pomegranate seeds	Gazpacho + 1 spelt and rye cracker + 1 tbsp aubergine dip	20g salted popcorn	Pastryless quiche + large mixed salad + 2 tsp dressing
Wednesday	1 poached egg + 1 slice wholemeal toast	1 spelt and rye cracker + 1 tbsp aubergine dip	Mushroom, spinach and tomato salad + 1 slice of wholemeal or granary bread with 1 tbsp cottage cheese	Savoury popcorn	100g roast chicken + brown rice pilaf + steamed green veg
Thursday	200ml Greek yoghurt + 50g blueberries	Banana	2 eggs, scrambled + 40g smoked salmon	1 spelt and rye cracker + 2 tbsp roasted red pepper and feta dip	Spanish chicken + 40g (raw weight) bulgur or wholegrain couscous
Friday	Smoothie made from 100g mango + 200ml milk + 5 tbsp Greek yoghurt	Apricot and pistachio power ball	Chicken and spelt salad	50g olives	Seafood tagine + 1 slice of wholemeal garlic bread + large green salad + 2 tsp dressing
Saturday	1 slice of wholemeal toast + ½ medium avocado + 1 rasher of grilled bacon + 1 poached egg	-	Mushroom, spinach and tomato salad + 1 wholemeal pitta	-	Chicken curry + 30g (raw weight) brown rice; + 1 poppadom
Sunday	Scrambled eggs (2 medium eggs and 1 tsp butter) + 40g smoked salmon	-	White bean and parsley soup	-	150g baked salmon + vegetable couscous; Fruits of the forest jelly

Week 5

	Breakfast	Snack	Lunch	Snack	Evening meal
Monday	Scrambled eggs (2 medium eggs and 1 tsp butter) + 1 slice wholemeal toast	Apple	Carrot, celeriac and coriander soup + 1 large slice of wholemeal bread; 100g plain yoghurt	20g savoury popcorn	Fish Provençal + steamed green veg + 1 wholemeal pitta
Tuesday	200ml Greek yoghurt + 50g raspberries	Apricot and pistachio power ball	Pumpkin and lentil salad; 1 orange	1 spelt and rye cracker + 1 tbsp roasted red pepper and feta dip	Pasta with ricotta and herb sauce; large green salad + 2 tsp dressing
Wednesday	2 tbsp sugar-free muesli + 200ml milk + handful of blueberries	100g pomegranate seeds	Gazpacho; 1 spelt and rye cracker + 2 tsp hummus	100g roasted chickpeas	Vietnamese chicken stir-fry + 30g (raw weight) brown rice
Thursday	2 tbsp sugar-free muesli + 100ml Greek yoghurt + 100ml milk	100g mango	Thai prawn salad; 100g plain yoghurt + handful of raspberries	20g savoury popcorn	Leek and ham gratin; large green salad + 2 tsp dressing + 1 tbsp croutons
Friday	1 slice wholemeal toast + ½ medium avocado + 1 slice of ham and 1 sliced tomato	3 Brazil nuts	½ avocado + 100g cooked peeled prawns + 1 mini wholemeal pitta	1 oatcake + 1 tbsp aubergine dip	Pork sliders and quick apple coleslaw + green salad + 2 tsp dressing
Saturday	Scrambled eggs (2 medium eggs and 1 tsp butter) + 40g smoked salmon + ½ wholemeal English muffin	-	Small can of tuna in oil + large mixed salad + 1 tsp oil	-	Greek lamb + green beans; Plain yoghurt + blackberries
Sunday	Veggie shakshuka	-	Lamb and barley soup	-	150g baked salmon + parsnip rösti + roasted Mediterranean vegetable salad; small fruit salad

Index

Thank you all

Huge love to the gang at Orion who've helped me put this new book together. Your energy and enthusiasm is contagious!!!!

Hugest thanks and hugs to Catherine Phipps for translating my likes and ideas into the best recipes (you read my mind) and for being on the end of the phone whenever I was feeling like a rookie! Andrew Hayes-Watkins is a total star and always makes the food look the best and me feel like a goddess. Loved our shoot days!!! Thanks to Anna Burges-Lumsden and her team for cooking all the dishes so expertly, to Loulou Clark, Helen Ewing and Olivia Wardle for their care in making every shot look mouth-wateringly tempting, and to Fiona Hunter for the expert nutritional advice. You're all fabulous. Thank you too to Paul Palmer-Edwards for great design.

As always, big thanks to Angie Smith, Michael Douglas and Cheryl Phelps-Gardiner for cleaning the flour off my face and making me look shamaze for the photos. To Amanda Harris for keeping everything on track with great charm and tact (and how do you look so goddamn gawjus while you are doing it?), and to Jinny Johnson for helping me with the words. Jinny... I love you. I hope you don't take offence because I mean this in the nicest possible way, but you are like my perfect mummy. Thank you.

And to my agents Rowan, Emily and Mary (a formidable posse of superwomen) for their constant support and advice and awesome kick buttness. Love you all. And, of course, massive thanks to Matthew and my children for their constant love and patience – and for eating everything I cook!

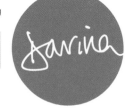